Safety for nurses and all medical staff at a hospital is essential. It is especially vital in today's society to know how to protect yourself. Matt's principles are simple, effective and easy to implement in high-stress situations. If you want to learn how to protect yourself and your loved ones, Matt's your guy.

Steph W, Nurse Anesthesiologist

Teaching today has a lot more responsibilities and fears associated with it — from disgruntled students to active shooters. Matt has helped me become a stronger person physically but also mentally, to aid me in my profession, no matter what the circumstances. His guidance on safety for myself and my students is simple and easy to remember. I pray that I never have to use any of the tools he has taught me, but if I do, I know I am prepared.

Rachel C, High-School Teacher

Being a mom of two little ones while also managing people all day in my job means you have to operate at your best at home and at work. Matt has given me simple tools to help me perform optimally throughout my day while keeping me safe if I am ever in a workplace-violence situation or need to protect my children.

Mindy T, CPA and Mother

Being a grandmother has its own set of challenges, but whether traveling with my grandchildren around town or alone across the globe, I can feel confident in my safety because of the tools and strategies Matt has given me. Thank you!

Andrea T, Grandmother

REINVENT
YOUR PERSONAL SAFETY
3 KEYS TO SUCCESSFUL SELF-PROTECTION FOR WOMEN

MATT TAMAS
FOREWORD BY SCOTT MANN
FORMER GREEN BERET & AUTHOR OF GAME CHANGERS

NEW YORK

NASHVILLE • MELBOURNE • VANCOUVER

REINVENT YOUR PERSONAL SAFETY

Published in New York, New York, by Morgan James Publishing. Morgan James is a trademark of Morgan James, LLC.
www.MorganJamesPublishing.com

The Morgan James Speakers Group can bring authors to your live event. For more information or to book an event visit The Morgan James Speakers Group at www.TheMorganJamesSpeakersGroup.com.

ISBN 978-1-68350-508-2 paperback
ISBN 978-1-68350-509-9 eBook
Library of Congress Control Number: 2017904595

Cover & Interior Design by:
Megan Whitney
Creative Ninja Designs
megan@creativeninjadesigns.com

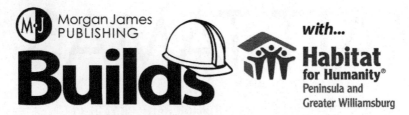

In an effort to support local communities, raise awareness and funds, Morgan James Publishing donates a percentage of all book sales for the life of each book to Habitat for Humanity Peninsula and Greater Williamsburg.

Get involved today! Visit
www.MorganJamesBuilds.com

CONTENTS

FOREWORD   XV

INTRODUCTION   1

Violence Against Women   3
The Problem of Self-Defense   4
Who is This Book For?   6
Who is This Book By?   7
3 Keys to Successful Self-Protection   8

1. PREPARE   11

Be Selfish   14
Take Responsibility   16
Defeat Limiting Beliefs   19
Don't "Fear" Fear   29
Your Reason to Prevail   32
Form Positive Habits   34
Summary   38

2. AVOID   41

Weigh Up Your Attacker   43
Trust Your Intuition   51
Be Alert   59
De-Select Yourself   70
Summary   76

3. ESCAPE   79

Defuse and De-Escalate   82
Precursors to Physical Attack   88
Your Combative Toolbox   89
Rely On Your Mind   118
Summary   120

CONCLUSION   123

YOUR PERSONAL SAFETY PLAN   124

BIBLIOGRAPHY   127

ACKNOWLEDGEMENTS   129

ABOUT THE AUTHOR
& QUANTUM PERSONAL SAFETY   131

FOREWORD

As a U.S. Army Green Beret, I've spent over two decades immersed in some of the most dangerous, trust-depleted places on earth. Violence has always been an unfortunate part of my career.

Along this journey, I've seen hundreds of programs and met dozens of so-called *experts* who address the issue of self-defense and personal protection. Some of them were better than others, but none of them ever struck me as game changers...until I met Matt Tamas.

In his book, *Reinvent Your Personal Safety*, Matt does far more than introduce *3 Keys to Successful Self-Protection for Women*. He provides a new way of thinking; a new way of acting...hell, he provides a whole new way of life for women living in a high-conflict world.

I don't follow theorists. I follow practitioners and leaders. Matt's book captures this entirely. The reasons are striking:

First, when it comes to changing the game of women's self-protection, it requires more than just understanding the dark act of exploitation. Matt Tamas LIVED it! He wrote this tough-minded book with the heartfelt empathy essential to taking on this sensitive issue.

Second, Matt knows how to fight back. He has significant combatives and protective training experience. The stuff he teaches is practical and immediately relevant—not in some climate controlled karate studio—but in the tricky corners of every-day life.

And third, Matt's approach is completely holistic. Matt gets beyond the one-dimensional physical aspects of fighting back and into the critical aspects of what should happen before an attack ever occurs. Matt is also highly accomplished in physical and spiritual resilience. Trust me, when it comes to thriving in a trust-depleted world, this holistic resilience is crucial to preventing and overcoming the myriad threats facing women today.

Finally, Matt writes this book not only as a warrior, but as a loving husband, and the father of two young girls. You better believe, that what Matt Tamas puts down on these pages, he lives into and teaches the most important ladies in his life - his wife and daughters! Just imagine what that kind of passion and focus could mean to your personal safety capacity.

Prepare.

Avoid.

Escape.

I've operated in the unforgiving crucible of combat for most of my adult life. The framework Matt puts forward in this book; is as powerful and immediately useful as any model I've ever used.

There is one more reason you should read Matt's book and take his coaching. I trained Matt myself. I've trained him many of the same skills Green Berets use against violent enemies, along with advanced leadership and inter-personal skills.

He is the best around. You're in great hands.

The world is changing fast, but the realm of self-protection is not. We need someone to lead us out of this stagnant place toward a world where women can chase their dreams without fear of their personal safety.

It's a noble mission in a dangerous time—and Matt Tamas will get us there.

Scott Mann
Former Green Beret and Author of Game Changers

INTRODUCTION

A lot of people don't really understand violence, manipulation, exploitation and abuse. I do, because I am a survivor of it.

When I was seventeen years old, I remember being shy, having low self-esteem and no confidence. I probably wasn't that much different from most seventeen-year-olds, to be honest. That's how old I was when I made a friend who changed my life. He offered me a job at a car dealership, a dream job for a car-crazy high-school student. In addition, he hired my friends and embedded himself in my inner circle. He used religion to bond with my parents, came to family events and, over the next year, this prominent business figure made me feel like a VIP. We went to bars, restaurants, sporting events, you name it. I felt like I was king of the world!

I was interested in male modeling at the time and when he asked me what I wanted to do, I told him. One day, right after my eighteenth birthday, he told me to meet him at his home. He said he knew someone who would get me into a book and he needed to take some photos. When I got there, he photographed me in the nude. The pictures didn't have my face in them. And I knew, then, that he was using me, that he had been manipulating me the whole time.

It changed my life. I felt dirty, betrayed and, above all, angry. I vowed from that day forward I would never be exploited or manipulated again.

And, at the same time, I became more aware of it when it was happening to other people.

As I moved through life, I made a key discovery when it came to the women that I got to know, and some that I dated. The majority of them had been physically, mentally or emotionally abused.

One woman I met after college, Michelle, was terrified of snakes – I mean absolutely terrorized by them. I asked her one day for the reason. What she told me has stayed with me for the rest of my life. You see, when she was a little girl, her parents hired a family friend to babysit her when they went out. Who better than a family friend, right? Well, as soon as her parents left, this "friend" would proceed to take her outside and stuff her down a dark well that was filled with snakes. The horror and torture she endured at his hands – someone her family trusted –lasted for years.

Now I have two daughters of my own. Savanna, who is five years old, is the spitting image of me right now. She has high self-esteem, incredible confidence and pride. Ashley is six. She is quiet, shy and has low self-esteem. She is an easy target for predators, just like I was. Just like the other victims I got to know were.

But she doesn't have to end up a victim. There are tools I can teach her to protect her from the enemy she may face one day. And I'm not talking about some random thug jumping out of the bushes – I'm talking about the real enemy who tries to gain your trust, who manipulates their way into your presence. Think about the women in your life who have been physically, psychologically or emotionally abused, who have been manipulated or exploited. Who was their attacker?

It's time for a paradigm shift in women's personal safety. We need to move away from teaching women martial arts moves to try to defend themselves against the unlikely random stranger jumping out at them. We need to move to a principle-driven system of self-protection that begins with training the mind, that recognizes the prevalent threat of the manipulative attacker, and that gives women a higher chance of keeping themselves safe.

I vow to help my daughters, especially Ashley, to be prepared later in life. Who is your Ashley? Is it your grandmother, mother, wife, aunt, sister, girl-friend, daughter—or is it you?

Violence Against Women

It goes almost without saying that the prevalence of violence against women is cause for concern in today's society. We only have to look at 2016's top news stories to see the trend, from Brock Turner's sexual assault of an un-conscious student on college campus to five men robbing Kim Kardashian West, bound and gagged, in her hotel suite. And these are just isolated head-line stories that got reported and got attention. On social media, writer Kelly Oxford's invitation to women to share their #firstassault garnered over a million responses in one evening. Many women hadn't previously told their story. Many never do, so the horrific statistics don't even do reality justice.

In 2013, the World Health Organization reported that, worldwide, thirty-five per cent of women had been subject to physical and/or sexual violence. And the statistics tell us that this is not generally perpetrated by the aggressive stranger on the street, but, for the most part, by intimate partners.

Twenty per cent of women have suffered sexual violence as children, the United Nations reporting that sixty million girls are assaulted on their way to school each year. In the United States alone, 1,615 women were murdered by men in 2013. The Department of Justice tells us that on average, there are 288,820 victims of rape and sexual assault in the country each year.

In the course of research for this book, I have heard so many terrible sto-ries—accounts of abuse of children by teachers and other pupils, tales of workplace violence at the hands of bosses and co-workers, accounts of date rape and domestic violence … Yet, when I ask people to picture their attacker, it's never someone they know, it's always someone who looks unkempt or rough, someone in the shadows. In reality, when women are attacked, it's more likely to be by someone they know or think they know – someone who looks normal.

And how do these people get close enough to cause harm? It's through manipulation, misdirection, being charming, wielding authority, building trust—playing on denial and apathy, and preying on those they identify as victims.

On a global scale, the United Nations cites World Bank data stating that women aged fifteen to forty-four are more at risk from rape and domestic violence than from cancer, car accidents, war and malaria.

But what can we do about it?

The Problem of Self-Defense

So can't you just take a weekend self-defense course and be done with it? No.

The problem with self-defense programs is a problem that is reflected in the way a lot of us live our lives—they are *reactive*.

Think about the way a lot of us go about things when it comes to making decisions. Generally, we only look to get a new job when we have lost the old one or after it has caused us untold stress. We often only look to work on weight-loss, fitness or nutrition once we become overweight and unfit or have health problems. We don't pre-empt the issues we're at risk of, often despite a lot of noise in the media that tells us we should. And when it comes to protecting ourselves, a lot of us only decide to consider our personal safety in a truly practical way once something has already happened to us or to someone close to home. We live life in a reactive way.

This is a big issue people face. They are caught up in victim mode. They live in an "effect" state, instead of being the cause in their own lives.

When it comes to personal safety, that's a problem.

If you've come to this book as a survivor of violence, I am so sorry. You are likely not alone. I've seen training classes where seventy per cent of the attendees are there because something has happened to them or someone close to them. Seventy per cent.

When it comes to training both survivors and those who haven't before been in a violent encounter, however, the approach is the same. It is *not* to teach people martial-arts-style self-defense, which is a reactive and technique-driven approach to facing an attacker.

Let me explain. When you're in a martial arts class, on the mats, not only are you likely in active attire, feeling lively, completely sober, and matched up with people who you know are never going to hurt you, but you're also taught moves that do not make sense in a real-life scenario. Making a roundhouse kick, or escaping a hold by using the right combination of moves while your forearm is in someone's grip, are techniques that require fine motor skills.

A motor skill is an action that involves using your muscles. Fine motor skills are those which involve more complicated movements, more muscles, and technique that requires a lot of practice to get right and is hard to replicate under stress (have you ever had to simply dial 911 under stress? It's incredibly difficult). And it's not just martial arts moves; flipping the top on a pepper spray, for example, involves fine motor skills. In contrast, gross motor tools, which I'll teach you when we get to the third part of the book, work with your body's natural reactions. They are larger actions that enhance your body's natural ability. We're talking about simple strikes; straightforward tools where the technicality of how you put them into practice doesn't actually matter – knowing the right targets matters. We're talking about moves that will be straightforward to put into practice if you're inebriated, regardless of what you're wearing, and in a space as small as a bathroom stall.

I actually have a problem even using the phrase self-defense. I never do when I'm coaching. Because, in my view, if you are defending, you are losing.

To prevail, you need to be on the offense. You need to take a proactive approach to the situations you find yourself in, and you need to take a proactive approach to personal safety.

This is what *self-protection* is about. In this book, I'm going to take you through a proactive approach to personal safety, one that isn't about honing technical moves or perfecting technique—it's about working with your body and your mind, considering realistic scenarios, and training you to take appropriate action. My job, as your personal safety coach, is to not only give you the tools to fight back during an assault, but also those to help you prevent yourself from being assaulted in the first place. The right action to take is often in advance of a likely violent encounter in order to *avoid it altogether*. The best way to protect yourself is avoiding the situation in which you are forced to *defend* yourself. We're going to talk about the different ways this is possible, as well as about the best way to handle yourself when violent confrontation simply cannot be avoided.

This means that you will be able to live your life at cause, rather than effect. It will give you control over your own safety. And this is something that is possible for everyone.

Who is This Book For?

When I ask women their fears, they're about being overcome by an attacker who's likely larger and stronger than them, in a dark parking lot, or in their own home at night, someone they "don't have a chance against." Women fear the utter helplessness of being overwhelmed, of being physically injured and raped, and of being psychologically scarred for life. As we've seen in the sad statistics, these are not groundless fears.

However, people assume a book on self-protection must be for the fit, flexible woman of a certain age (not too old but not too young), who can train in martial-arts-style combat and hold her own on the mats if she learns certain techniques. And this just isn't true.

This book is for the high-school girl, for the grandmother, for the young professional, for the working mother—anyone who is willing to overcome their limiting beliefs about what they're capable of and key into what self-protection is really about. In reality, knowledge of the appropriate action to take in any given situation is worth scores more than athleticism.

This is training that you can do in your living room. You do not *need* to go to a gym. You do not *need* to go to a self-defense class and learn correct punching technique. When we get to the physical part, we'll talk about enhancing the body's natural abilities and turning them into appropriate action. But way before and above the physical tools, we're going to talk about the things we can learn to do day-to-day that change the probability of our encountering a violent physical attack, and increase our chances of survival.

Mentally, it's about taking a proactive approach and being at cause rather than effect; emotionally, it's about understanding fear as an asset and using our beliefs to help us prevail; physically, it's about engaging appropriately and focusing on the right targets—and we can train ourselves to do all of these things, whatever our age, appearance or athletic ability.

So whether you're a fourteen-year-old high-school student or an eighty-five-year-old grandmother, it's worth reading on. You are capable of protecting yourself.

Who is This Book By?

My path to becoming an expert in personal safety began nearly twenty years ago.

After becoming a Certified Strength & Conditioning Specialist, I turned my focus on the field of self-protection. I completed multiple personal safety certifications under coach Tony Torres, who developed the Functional Edge System of self-protection, while studying the best teaching principles and training programs around the world with a multitude of instructors. I incorporated everything I learned into my own consulting business and have been coaching people in personal safety ever since, from lawyers, athletes and entrepreneurs to CEOs and moms.

The research and training didn't stop there, with my passion for teaching people the best way to protect themselves only becoming deeper. I undertook mentorships with leadership expert Scott Mann, a retired Green Beret, and executive coach Peter Sage, a renowned public speaker and expert in personal development.

The idea for this book for women has grown as my family has grown. As husband to a woman who is beautiful both inside and out, and father to three beautiful children, I've become aware of the void in our society in terms of what is being taught to women with regard to their personal safety.

Bringing together everything I've learned throughout my personal safety career, I've founded QuantumPersonalSafety.com and The Quantum Academy to provide woman all around the world access to effective and practical personal safety instruction from their own home.

3 Keys to Successful Self-Protection

The principles I present here are a template to success. They make up a holistic approach to self-protection that allows you to form your own personal safety plan. There are three key elements to apply, which I'll take you through in the three parts to this book:

1. **Prepare:** Ninety per cent of training yourself to handle violence is mental. Survival is about mindset. In this part of the book, we'll talk about combating apathy and denial, reprogramming your mind, and tapping into your reason to prevail.

2 **Avoid:** The best way to prevail against an attacker is to avoid a violent encounter altogether. In this part of the book, we'll talk about how to weigh up your attacker, recognize a threat, and learn the arts of being alert and de-selecting yourself.

3 **Escape:** Our primary aim in every situation is getting away and reaching safety. If we can't avoid a violent encounter, then this means engaging—engaging verbally to defuse and de-escalate a situation where this is possible, and, if all else fails, engaging physically and in the appropriate way to escape from harm. In this part of the book, we'll cover the verbal and physical tools you can practice to keep you safe.

Throughout, I'm going to be taking you through strategy, tactics and tools. Strategy is your plan of action. It involves preparation ahead of time to get a result. Tactics are your physical manifestation of strategy. They involve efficient use of thought and action. Tools are your mental or physical means of accomplishing a task or achieving your purpose.

Your beliefs need to be aligned with your strategy, tactics and tools or you'll end up in conflict. This is something we'll look at in Part 1. The principles I'm going to teach you are your foundation for success.

As we go through these key principles, you'll find examples and exercises to help you engage with the material. At the end of the day, it's not about theory; it's about performance. I'm going to teach you how to perform when you need to protect yourself. I'll demonstrate the practical application of the guidance in hypothetical and real-life scenarios. Where relevant, I'll direct you to any external resources, such as training videos, at QuantumPersonalSafety. com. This is where you'll find a community of like-minded people committed to personal safety and the connection of heart, mind and soul.

So let's begin!

PREPARE

'It is the mind that must first be properly prepared,
the mind which controls the hands, arms, eyes, and ears.'

GAVIN DE BECKER

Sarah was a client who came to me for personal safety instruction. She was a middle-aged woman who worked as an executive assistant in an accounting firm, and she had been the victim of workplace violence at the end of a Christmas party held at her offices, where a colleague had accosted and sexually assaulted her when they were alone.

When I sat down with Sarah to talk about her experiences and her beliefs, and to talk about the pre-attack elements and the importance of preparation, she was surprised. She had obviously expected some talking about and reliving of her experience, but she had been expecting, and hoping, to move right into what she considered the learning part of it all—where she'd find out how to pull the right moves in a similar situation that would mean she escaped. The problem with this type of thinking is that no one has the perfect answer to what you have to do in the moment—it all depends. An instructor who plays armchair quarterback, judging your actions and dictating what you should do, is an instructor you need to fire ASAP. There are too many variables at stake for someone to know what will work in one moment in time. That's why being prepared with principles is the answer – it gives you the tools to succeed no matter the variables involved. Techniques limit you; principles make you limitless.

When we think about being attacked, we automatically think of the physical aspect, and everyone wants to learn the secret move or technique that will have them overpowering an assailant. However, in reality, ninety per cent of personal safety is the mental aspect.

I talked to Sarah about her offices, where the attack took place, and about her co-worker. I asked her what she felt in the moments before the attack took place, and she said she felt uncomfortable and "funny." Delving into this, we identified what might have contributed to that feeling. Her attacker had stood a bit too close for comfort, invading her personal space, and had not taken note of her leaning back, signaling that she didn't want him so near. I asked her why she didn't act on those feelings and that was when I learned what she believed. She believed she could never really be in danger in her office – a place she saw as secure and one she knew well. She believed she could never really be in danger if there were other people close by – even if they were separated by a wall. She believed she was so much older than him that he couldn't *seriously* be propositioning her– not taking into account that sexual assault is far more about power and control than the act of sex, and that age difference is no barrier to attack. She believed she would never really be at risk from anyone she worked with – her unconscious assumption was that anyone who qualified to work for her company must be a "good" person and that they wouldn't do something that would obviously have damaging consequences for their career.

Sarah vaguely knew the co-worker in question, and he was friendly with people she was friendly with, so she felt like she should be polite even if he was making her uncomfortable. Logic and social convention demanded that she think through the situation and find excuses, rather than trusting her gut and immediately employing her mind to achieve her escape. Humans are actually the only species that do this. Animals act on their instincts! Instead of acting on the obvious, Sarah looked for the logical. She talked herself out of feeling scared and acting on that feeling. And that was entirely down to her mind.

When she realized she was truly in danger, she froze. She said her mind went completely blank. Then she screamed. But either no one heard – the music was still blaring next door – or people heard and did their own thinking, excusing and dismissing. Sarah admitted that she might have been more alert to the signs of danger if she'd been outside on the street in the dark being accosted by a stranger, but she truly didn't believe this could be happening to her. She didn't know what to do. She panicked. He was bigger than her and stronger than her and younger than her, and she didn't know any "self-defense" moves, so she immediately saw that she didn't really have a chance.

She couldn't have been further from the truth. And that was the first thing that I taught her.

The mind always leads the body. There's no point me teaching you anything if you secretly think that, in a real-life situation, it won't make a difference. The first thing I had to do with Sarah was reverse her thinking about what self-protection is and where it begins. It doesn't begin in the street; it begins in your brain.

You need to think of this book as the computer software you need to update your mind with practical and simple knowledge to help stack the deck in your favor when it comes to a life or death situation.

Yes, you can do things to be prepared physically, and I will give you those tools in Part 3, but I can't stress enough the difference that preparing yourself mentally makes. A person who hasn't trained their mind when it comes to personal safety will probably freeze with fear. You'll be out-numbered before the conflict even begins, because you'll be fighting your negative mindset as well as your attacker.

The only thing you can control, in any aspect of life, is yourself. So it's you who needs to take on the responsibility of being prepared mentally. This key element of self-protection is about being able to rely on your mind – your primary weapon. It is about understanding that you are the first responder in any situation, and how you respond is ninety per cent down to mindset. The number one thing you can control is your own mind.

In this part of the book, we'll address how to set your mind up for success – combating apathy and denial, and defeating limiting beliefs that might hold you back from protecting yourself.

Be Selfish

The first thing I'm going to ask you to do is be selfish.

Let me clarify: when I tell you to be selfish, I'm talking about taking care of *you* first. It's only by taking care of yourself that you can help others.

Just think about when you are on a flight and the flight attendants take you through the safety demonstration. If there is a loss in cabin pressure, air masks will drop down in front of you. And what do the flight attendants always say? They tell you to put the mask over your own face *first*. They say that by taking care of yourself first, you'll be better able to help your loved ones next.

But it seems like the more selfish act, right? Why can't you just slip the mask over the child beside you first – the more "unselfish" thing to do? Isn't that normally what we do – put the children first?

The thing is, hypoxia (oxygen deprivation) can set in incredibly rapidly. It may come with warning signs: shortness of breath, dizziness, blurry vision and mental confusion. But at higher altitudes, depressurization and unconsciousness can occur within a few seconds. You can't help anyone else if you pass out in the process. It's more efficient to take care of your needs first so you can assist children and other passengers with your full faculties intact, however selfish the act of saving yourself first might seem.

Take an example in a broader context. Imagine someone running around here, there and everywhere, so focused on their loved ones and helping everyone else that they lose sight of taking care of themselves in the process.

They wake up early in the morning in order to get the kids ready and get them off to school. They make sure that the kids have time for breakfast, but they don't have time to grab something themselves. Then they hit traffic and have to get themselves to work. Work is busy, so they don't grab more than some coffee and, later, takeout to eat at their desk. They work late, then hit traffic, then make it home. Their partner's picked up the kids and sorted them out with dinner, but the kids still need help with their homework. Then a colleague calls, needing a favor or an ear to bend, and they don't have the heart to say they don't have time to do what's asked of them. They don't eat till late, then only get to watch a little television before bed and the whole cycle starting again.

They make unhealthy food choices, don't make time for exercise, become overweight, don't make time for relaxation (that would be selfish), and the list goes on ... Life can spiral out of control. Focusing on everything and everyone apart from yourself, it's easy to neglect your diet and exercise, sacrifice your sleep and lose touch with your friends and personal interests. You might consider yourself the most selfless person around, but what do you think happens next?

You become stressed. And stress can cause a variety of problems, internal and external, including physical ailments and chronic illness. You turn into the one who needs help, and your ability to help others is forfeited.

Even though you spent all this time refusing to be selfish, it backfires, because then you require others to be selfless in order to look after you. And you're in no position to look after them in return.

Being selfish in this context is one of the most important things you can do, not just for your own health and wellbeing but also that of others.

It's the same thing when it comes to your personal safety. If you go day by day, ignoring the risks and not investing the time in learning how to protect yourself because, subconsciously, you think it's only you at stake and focusing that time and energy on yourself would be selfish, then you have to think again. If you are being attacked, you better be in a position to fight for your life, with the chances stacked in your favor. Put yourself first, even if the idea seems selfish. Put the mask on yourself before doing anything else. You are a VIP, and your family, friends and loved ones need you.

An attack on you is an attack on them. The ripple effect would be huge if something were to happen to you. Imagine the effects on your children if you're injured so badly you can't look after them. Imagine the effects psychologically, trying to be a friend to someone when you've undergone massive trauma. Imagine the psychological effects on your partner and everyone around you, who know what you've been through and are hurting because of it. Imagine the normal life you led before being at an end, and the normal lives of the ones around you, because of a single moment in time that could go a different way if you prepared.

So start with being selfish. Admit your worth to yourself. Part of preparation for overcoming violence is accepting that you need to take care of yourself first. It doesn't take that much time and, with minimal investment, you get a huge reward. You protect what's most valuable – you!

Take Responsibility

Too many people live in a world of apathy. Despite all the violence in the world, when it comes to the idea that they themselves will encounter violence, they live in denial. Too many people are reactive when it comes to personal safety, and only think about their self-protection when something happens to them or something happens close to home. Instead, we need to take a proactive approach to violence – don't act once something has already happened, when it's too late to avoid it or deal with it.

One of the greatest advantages that an attacker has over you is your attitude of apathy around keeping yourself safe.

A victim who lives a life of apathy goes through life unconcerned, thinking to themselves that violence doesn't occur in their city, their town, their neighborhood, or on their street. Most victims living a life of apathy ask themselves during an attack, "Why me?" They think, "I can't believe this is happening."

Victims are usually in complete denial that violence will ever happen to them. I personally know a lot of people who live in affluent areas and leave their doors unlocked, even when away on vacation, because they think crime doesn't happen in their town. Think for a moment. How many people do you know who talk about crime as if it only happens in other towns or cities, not theirs?

If you choose to live your life making excuses, and rationalizing or justifying things rather than taking control and changing them, then you are living a life in denial. You *must* change how you think about violence. This will automatically help stack the deck in your favor. Personal safety is about accepting that violence does exist and that it can happen to anyone regardless of age, gender, wealth, social status, and so on.

This is not to say that you should live your life expecting to be attacked, peering around every corner or bush. But it is about accepting that attacks can happen, so you can be more prepared. I'm not telling you to be paranoid; I'm telling you to be *present*.

In personal safety, one of the most important lessons you can learn is to take responsibility for yourself. In personal security, there is a saying: "You Are It."

You have to know that relying on the police, first responders, your spouse, friends, neighbors or anyone else is a recipe for disaster. *You* are the first responder when it comes to violence.

There are two things I want to talk about in relation to this. The first is emergency service response times. You cannot afford to wait without taking action, holding on for the police to show up, if you are under threat,. You don't control how long it will take for them to get to you. You don't control what your attacker does in the meantime.

The second thing I want to talk about is the bystander effect. This is where the presence of others around someone actually discourages them from taking action and intervening in an emergency situation. This concept was first talked about in the mainstream after the murder of a woman named Kitty Genovese in 1964. Her rape and stabbing outside her apartment building was witnessed by several dozen bystanders. They did nothing to help her. They didn't even call the police.

Why was this? Some said they didn't realize they were witnessing a crime. Others assumed that someone else had already called the authorities. The psychologists called it perceived diffusion of responsibility, and the effect of social influence. The more people around, the less likely someone is to take responsibility upon themselves to act. And individuals in a group take their cue from those around them. Onlookers in this case concluded from the inaction of their neighbors that their action wasn't required.

The existence of the phenomenon has been backed up time and again by clinical study and by real-life events. The film *The Accused* tells the true-life story of the gang rape of Cheryl Araujo in a bar – where onlookers failed to help or call for aid. In 2009, up to twenty bystanders witnessed the rape of a fifteen-year-old girl outside a homecoming dance without intervening or calling the police. In both cases, some witnesses even cheered or laughed.

I even heard about the bystander effect happening to one of my friends in a park as a young teen, long before I'd ever come across the term. She was accosted by a group of kids and punched in the face. The park wasn't empty – there were plenty of people about – but nobody did anything. Not any of the adults, not any of the kids. They just watched it happen. Watched her face start bleeding. Watched her run away. Watched the others run after her.

People aren't always conscious that their first instinct is to deny or shift responsibility. But there's nothing stopping *you* from being conscious of it, and choosing to take responsibility for what unfolds. We might think that people being around will be a deterrent to violence, or at least will mean more people to help if something happens, but the psychology of apathy means we can't rely on the logic here.

You cannot rely on outside help. You cannot pause because the best course of action seems to be waiting for someone else to come to the rescue, even if you're aware that there are other people around, even if you think the police are on their way. You can't necessarily count on them. And in an attack, minutes, even seconds, count.

Don't live your life in victim mode, denying your self-worth. And don't become a victim because you think someone else is going to save you. You need to give yourself permission to act. The only person that you can rely on 100 per cent of the time is yourself. So take responsibility for yourself and your own safety.

Defeat Limiting Beliefs

The idea that you can reprogram your mind is probably one of the most important concepts you will ever learn in terms of personal safety.

Most people are experts at using their mind to imagine negative outcomes. They could see some amazing results in their lives if they used their mind to pursue positive thoughts the same way they do negative ones. They don't realize that it's possible to reprogram your mind and replace the negative default program. It takes the same amount of energy to produce negative or positive thoughts!

For most people, all that's limiting them is their beliefs. Whether you think you can or you think you can't – it actually doesn't matter. Both trains of thought are correct. If you think you can't do something, you won't. If you think you can do something, you will.

Now, in order to be able to change them, it's important to first understand what beliefs are and how they are created.

A belief is your attitude toward something. It is a statement of "truth" you have created for yourself, usually through taking on the belief of someone else. It's a thought to which you have attached a deep-rooted feeling.

For example, a belief could be that talking to strangers is bad. You might believe this because of years of repetition – your parents, teachers and relatives will have beaten it into your mind that talking to strangers is bad and your mind has taken up the chant. It's become an attitude associated with strong emotions.

In reality, if I don't know you, should I automatically assume you are bad? Think about it; despite what we've all been taught, a stranger isn't automatically a danger. A stranger can help save your life. Meanwhile, as the statistics show, it's the people we haven't categorized as "danger" who often pose the biggest threat.

It's important to understand this because other people and things don't really create your beliefs. You are the only person who can create a belief. And if you have the power to create it, you have the power to control it.

Lots of information gets presented to us through our senses; it all goes into our brain where it is processed and a belief is created. Your brain truly doesn't know the difference between a real and imagined experience. All your brain has to refer to when it comes to making decisions about anything is the information that it receives. It's what you do inside your brain that really matters.

Let's use my wife as a real-life example. She might get mad at me, but it's for a good cause, right? Now, my wife has had a fear of public speaking since college, because she once had a bad experience. She would still talk about how much she hated speaking in front of large groups of people many years later.

That was due to her experience. The information in her mind was that she gave a talk in front of some other students and it didn't go well. What came next were the feelings and emotions that your brain releases when you experience an event. Let's say you process the information and tell yourself that it was bad, scary and nerve-wracking, as most people would.

When you've processed the event you've experienced, you start to feel the associated emotions run through you. The result is that the mind associates speaking in front of groups of people with the negative emotions running through you, such as embarrassment, shame and fear.

However, in reality, an event is just an event. It's your beliefs about the event that peg it as bad or good. You could have 1,000 people witness an event and possibly have 1,000 different beliefs about the outcome of that event.

The experience itself doesn't really matter; that is just the information going to your brain. What matters is what happens with the information once it gets to your brain.

The first thing my wife did was categorize standing up in front of a classroom and speaking as scary and bad, which allowed her body to feel those negative emotions. What she did was create the root of a belief in her brain.

So, for her, the root of the belief is that public speaking results in her feeling extreme nervousness, embarrassment and fear. Every time she thinks about public speaking or tells anyone her feelings about it, she replays that negative experience over and over in her mind, and reinforces the belief.

Sometimes, it only takes one negative experience to form a limiting belief.

Take a moment and reflect on this point. Can you think of any of your own limiting beliefs? Can you trace them back to their roots?

What about when it comes to your personal safety?

Imagine two women who have equal physical skills but differing belief systems about their abilities. The woman who believes she will prevail against her attacker will. The woman who doesn't believe in herself has the odds greatly stacked against her.

The most important piece of advice here is that everything must be aligned. What alignment means for personal safety is that your belief system correlates to your mental and physical abilities.

The mind navigates the body. If you don't believe you can prevail against your attacker, you won't − no matter how much knowledge you attain or skills you possess. Having limiting beliefs and self-doubt will block you when it's time for you to take action and prevail against an attacker, so you need to work through such beliefs.

Let's look at some examples.

LIMITING BELIEFS

- Someone in a position of trust must be a good person. I am not at risk from them.

- If someone's decided they want to harm me, I won't be able to do anything about it.

- The best course of action is always not to resist and just hope not to get hurt.

- It will never happen to me.

- People mostly get attacked by strangers.

- All I have to do is scream. Someone will help.

- I am too old and unfit to fight back and get away from someone trying to harm me.

- I can't strike first; I'll get into trouble. Being struck gives me permission to strike.

- Women who learn self-protection lose their femininity.

- Nothing will make a difference. I cannot fight off someone bigger and stronger than me.

These are limiting beliefs that will hold you back from doing whatever you can to protect yourself. Take, for example, the common idea that if you are old and/or unfit, you won't be able to get away from an attacker. You may have read about such a scenario in the news more than once – the strong preying on the weak. Or you may have seen someone older unable to do a certain task and formed the judgment accordingly. However, holding such a belief can cause you to give up the fight before it's even begun. It is defeatist. It doesn't take into account that there are principles that can be put into play in close quarters regardless of age or fitness level. Feeling like your actions won't make any difference may cause you to freeze and not take any action at all. But you always have options, and only action will save you.

Just by challenging such beliefs you can begin to turn the tables and align yourself with what you *can* do, rather than becoming their prisoner.

You need to have a conversation with yourself ahead of time, in a relaxed state, on whether you are mentally prepared to fight back if a situation ever becomes physical. You have to be prepared ahead of time and know that you will do whatever it takes to survive — no matter what the cost.

Can you impose physical harm on your attacker? Can you palm-strike him to his face or groin? Can you gouge out an attacker's eye? Crush his throat? Rip or tear an ear off?

You have to believe that you have it in you to cause physical harm, even if that means killing an attacker if your life is on the line. You must survive. You must believe you can.

This is the really important part about understanding your mind and changing your mindset. Each and every time you replay something in your mind, your brain takes it for a "real" experience. Whether it is happening in the physical world or only in your head, it is no different. This is how the information is processed.

It's like walking the same way through the snow over and over again — eventually you will make a path that becomes the quickest and easiest route to follow.

Most people don't understand how their mind works and let themselves fall into this trap as a result. However, once you understand the way your mind works, it means you can trick your brain. You can completely reverse limiting beliefs by manipulating how your brain works.

To put it simply, if you can imagine something inside your mind, your mind will assume it is real. By controlling how your emotions respond to the thought, you will start developing a belief about something, even if this runs counter to a belief you already hold. Through a process of repetition, you can replace the old belief with a new one.

My wife reprogrammed her mind when it came to public speaking. She went over and over the association of being relaxed, confident and even ecstatic about public speaking, to the point where the idea of speaking in front of people elicited a positive emotional response. She strengthened the association between public speaking and positive emotions instead of negative ones. By applying these tools, she has been able to reverse her limiting belief.

It helps to have "real" experiences to reinforce this training, but the beauty is that you can do this without them. This is excellent news for your personal safety.

You can start by creating a positive belief that an attack or confrontation can end with a positive outcome. We'll look at the steps you can take to do this in the next section. The main thing is that you associate this belief with positive emotions such as triumph and relief. If an attack ever does happen to you, you already have a mental blueprint where you prevail.

Let's talk about this in terms of visualization.

Positive Visualization

It's been well documented that a lot of famous athletes use mental training more than physical training because it allows them to train perfectly at all hours of the day. Take Dr. JoAnn Dahlkoetter's work with Olympic athletes as a sports psychologist and performance coach. She speaks of an Olympic speed skater she worked with and how visualization helped her to succeed. Dahlkoetter describes every step of the imagery the skater used, which incorporated all of her five senses into the experience: feeling her forefoot pushing off the track, hearing her skating splits, seeing herself surge ahead of her competition. Going through the elements of the race over and over again using mental training techniques meant she set a new American record at the Olympic Trials.

In the same way, Olympic skiers will go over the perfect run in their mind. They know every turn and how they will feel at each turn. Sometimes, on TV, they will actually show you the racer going through his/her mental training before the actual event – it's pretty cool to watch. They can see and feel themselves flying down the mountain as fast as they can possibly go and finishing a flawless race. They can tell you about the feel of the snow and the terrain at any point on the course.

Do you think that is the only time they are using visualization? Athletes imagine success twenty-four hours a day. Practice really does make permanence. The important thing to note is that it has to be the right kind of visualization.

A lot of people speak about using visualization for success, but very few people really teach the different types of visualizing that people do on a day-to-day basis.

Most of the visualizing that people do is useless, because it is more like daydreaming. The mind wanders aimlessly with no direction or consistency; it's more of a distraction than anything productive. Daydreaming about something gets you nowhere; it just wastes valuable time.

Purposeful visualization is the form that most personal development gurus teach their students. However, in reality, it's very ineffective as well, and only slightly better than daydreaming. The only difference between daydreaming and purposeful visualization is that, with the latter, you may look at a picture on a wall, in your wallet or in your bathroom on a daily basis and think about it 24/7, instead of just letting your mind wander with no visual to guide it.

To develop a truly helpful visualization technique, you need to do more.

The future that is created depends on where your attention goes. For visualization to truly create the outer world you envision, you must be fully engaged in your heart, mind and soul. That means your psychological, emotional and physical self all have to be one – completely aligned with each other.

This example will help you in the arena of personal safety. Throughout the process, imagine yourself taking action in full detail. At each step, engage your emotions – experience how you feel at every point.

1. **Create an environment.** (Picture yourself after work in a parking lot, or walking to your car after shopping. You could be out on a first date.)

2. **Create a frame of mind.** (You're exhausted from a long day, stressed out, or distracted.)

3. **Think of a potential situation.** (Someone wants to ambush you to steal your valuables or rape you while you are on a date.)

4. **Develop the scenario.** (You are walking to your car; a guy comes up to you and alarms go off in your gut. Or you're back at your date's apartment and he's pressuring you to stay.)

5. **Create a confrontation.** (Picture yourself getting attacked, or your date starting to get forceful with you. Imagine how you would move.)

6. **Slow it down.** (Observe the strikes and reactions from your attacker.)

7. **Create a response.** (See yourself attacking the attacker.)

8. **Create an outcome.** (Enact how you overcome your attacker and escape.)

We'll revisit exercises like this in the next two parts of the book, once I've gone through some of the avoidance tools, verbal tools and physical tools you should learn. These will help you to flesh out the final steps in different scenarios with appropriate action.

The main point here is to really feel the emotions. If you don't feel the emotions within your body, then this process won't work. Your brain won't have anything to attach the experience to.

If your mind attaches a bad emotion or emotions to a thought, it will remember and tell you not to do something. If it has good associations, it will remember this too and make you want to proceed.

All the mind wants is more positive stuff, so it is absolutely crucial to feel positive emotions when you picture your success. Once you have imagined an outcome and it has gone really well, the next thing you want is to really *feel* the emotions.

What emotions would you feel after thwarting an attack? Excited, confident, happy to be safe? Let the feelings trickle through your body and then repeat the process over and over again.

When you imagine taking an action, the positive outcome that goes with it is attached to the proper emotions that follow the outcome. Your mind essentially associates that action with a positive outcome and emotion.

The more you do this, the stronger that belief will be. This means it will be easier to take action if the situation arises in real life.

You won't ignore a threatening feeling because it's associated with someone in a position of trust. You won't submit, thinking that you're less likely to get hurt. You won't eschew responsibility for your survival, only screaming and waiting for someone to come. You won't hesitate before striking merely because you haven't yet been struck yourself. You won't freeze, deciding that there's nothing you can do to get away if someone bigger is assaulting you. Freezing is the response to having no options, but when it comes to your personal safety, you ALWAYS have options.

By revisiting specific limiting beliefs and putting them into different scenarios where this belief is upended, we can entirely reprogram our mind with new beliefs.

We can turn these new beliefs into positive affirmations.

Positive Affirmations

Forming positive affirmations is sometimes called constructive imagination. When you construct your affirmations, you want to identify exactly what it is that you want to develop and strengthen, then attach positive emotions to it.

So how do you write and use them? First, make sure your affirmations are specific and in the present tense. The most important point when constructing them is to make sure you write them as if you are already achieving the result. I suggest not having more than ten in practice at one time, and not making them too long – no longer than a couple of lines.

Your affirmations should be practiced upon waking and right before you fall asleep at night, because that is when your mind is quiet and relaxed.

Crucially, make sure you don't just read them. You have to feel deep inside that you have already achieved the affirmation.

Here are a couple of examples in regard to your personal safety:

POSITIVE AFFIRMATIONS

- If someone decides they want to harm me, I know I can stop them.

- I can resist against an attacker.

- If I'm in a violent encounter, I don't have to wait for help. I can help myself

- I am young enough to fight back in an attack.

- I am old enough to fight back in an attack.

- I am fit enough to prevail against an attacker.

- I can get away from someone trying to harm me.

- I can strike first in order to escape an attacker.

- I can fight off someone bigger and stronger than me.

- I have the knowledge and tools to keep myself and my loved ones safe.

Write down your own set of affirmations. Go through them as many times as you need to throughout your day, making sure not to skip the two most important times of day – before falling asleep and upon waking.

Don't "Fear" Fear

Part of training your brain involves looking at different emotions and how they cause you to act. We've already covered apathy and denial, but now for the big one. Fear.

Here is my take on fear: Fear is here to *help* you. Gavin de Becker, an expert on managing violence, goes so far as to call fear a gift.

I am not referring here to unnecessary fears that manifest as worry and anxiety, which are created in your mind. Worrying about something in the future and building up anxiety can be controlled in our minds. I'm talking here about the difference between being afraid about how a job interview might go tomorrow – and a very real fear about someone attacking you and causing you harm.

True fear is the ultimate signal from your intuition. It is the emotion that drives you to survive when your life is on the line. This fear triggers a biological reaction to take place to help you either flee or fight.

Let me break this biological reaction down. It is often called the fight or flight response. In a stressful situation, your body's sympathetic nervous system activates physiological changes in the body. These start with the amygdala and the hypothalamus, which are parts of the brain. The amygdala triggers the hypothalamus, and, in turn, the pituitary gland, the master gland at the base of the brain, is stimulated. This produces hormones that travel through the body and control its functions. In this case, the adrenocorticotropic hormone is released, which stimulates cortisol production, and the adrenal gland is stimulated, which means that epinephrine, better known as adrenaline, is released. While the hormone cortisol increases blood pressure and blood sugar, and suppresses the immune system, adrenaline increases blood flow to muscles and the contraction rate of the heart.

What this is all in aid of is a massive boost of energy. In terms of your body's capabilities, this increases strength and speed for more effective fighting or running. Not only do your heart rate and muscle tension increase, but also your blood clotting function, in order to prevent excessive blood loss if you're injured.

This means that you can look at fear in a different way. It doesn't have to be this negative feeling that means something bad is happening. Fear is a good thing, as it is there to assist our survival. So reprogram your mind to recognize it for what it is.

You can look at fear as an alarm and as fuel.

When looked at as an alarm, it is your built-in security system. It is there to help you survive. This alarm can go off without you necessarily having identified the cause of the fear, in which case you need to automatically and immediately look for danger by broadening your vision, while concentrating on exhaling to help lower your heart rate.

When I talk about broadening your vision, I mean extending your external focus. As we go about our lives, whatever we're engaged in, we often have narrow vision. We only look at the things we consider important to what we're doing. Rather than broad focus, we often have critical focus directed on our immediate task. This may be scrolling through our phone as we walk down the street, meaning we don't observe what else is going on along or across the street. If we're on public transport with friends, our critical focus is generally taken up with them and the conversation we're having. We might not even notice the other people in the space around us, except to casually observe whether it's crowded or empty.

In contrast, broadening your vision is about taking the time to observe the wider environment around you. When we treat fear as an alarm, we immediately extend our focus and go on the alert for danger.

As fuel, fear is designed to get your body moving; either fighting or fleeing. It's what you need to get going and protect yourself when you need to most. This is your body's way of preparing you for survival by increasing its performance capabilities.

You need to use the hormones that the fear response injects into your system. As explained, these increase your performance physically and mentally, and, therefore, increase the effectiveness of the action you take. Without an understanding of the mental and physical responses that take place, fear may work against you by causing confusion and panic in the moment. But by knowing what is really going on inside your body, you can use it to your advantage.

When you feel that increased heart rate, the blood pounding in your ears, the slight nausea that comes with a hit of adrenaline – *know* that your body's systems are pumping you with energy. *Know* that it means that if you choose to run, you will be faster than normal, faster than you might think is possible. Know that it means that if you choose to strike, you will be stronger than normal, hitting harder than you ever have. Knowing these facts will help reinforce your positive beliefs about your capability to overcome violence in the moment. And as we've discussed, if you believe something is possible, if you truly believe it, the odds are stacked in your favor.

So don't "fear" fear. Use it. It's your ally. It's going to make it easier for you to prevail.

Your Reason to Prevail

Next, I want to address something that overrides virtually everything else when it comes to successful self-protection. We've gone through some ways we can make it easier to prevail by altering our mindset, our very belief system. But we haven't addressed the biggest question: Why? Why do you *have* to win?

Put simply, in order to overcome an aggressor, you have to tap into your reason to prevail. This is probably the most important performance enhancement tool you will ever have available to you at any given moment. This is your true motivation to overcome violence.

When a threat arises, this reason to prevail is the spark that ignites you into taking action. It is the trigger that gets you moving. In essence, it is your real reason to live.

For some people, it will be their children; for others, their boyfriend/girlfriend or husband/wife. It might be the work you are doing in the world or the legacy you won't get a chance to leave if you are harmed. It is your passion – your will to survive. Whatever it is, it is something so dear to you that it causes you to switch from prey to predator instantly.

It's this switch that changes a response from "How can this be happening to me? I don't know what to do!" to "How do I overcome this? What is my best option?" You don't want to be frozen in disbelief; you want to be intent on action. This is your purpose, your "why," the spark that ignites the jet fuel and gets your butt into gear. This is what will drive you to fight from the very core of your being.

Please don't underestimate the power of this part of yourself. Time and time again, people will go to the defense of others such as friends, family and children before they will protect themselves. There are hundreds of stories, from that of Angela Cavallo, who lifted a car that had collapsed off the jacks on top of her son with her bare hands, to that of Maureen Lee, who attacked and fended off a cougar that had pounced on her three-year-old daughter.

As we've discussed, in a situation where violence is present, you have to be selfish. If you are being physically attacked, you must use the same thought process and trigger the same emotions as you would watching someone very dear to you being assaulted.

If someone tries to stop you from getting home to your child, imagine your child is there and under direct threat. You have to save yourself to save them.

An attacker doesn't just harm you; they harm everyone who loves and cares about you. They harm your potential, your very future – everything you could go on to be. If that isn't motivation enough to fight back, then I don't know what is.

Here are some tips to help you figure out your reason to prevail:

YOUR REASON TO PREVAIL

- It must be personal.

- It will be something or someone you are passionate about.

- It has to be important to you NOW – in the present, not something from the past.

- It is what makes you tick. Deep down, it makes you who you are.

- It is a trigger. The thought of losing it is what will get you angry enough to attack your attacker, rather than acting like prey, overtaken by fear.

- It isn't logical; it's emotional – something that rips you at your core, deep in your heart and soul.

You need to take some time to uncover this part of yourself. It might be a very simple answer, but, again, you need to really think about it and engage your emotions at the same time. In a life-or-death situation, the last thing you want to do is freeze. You want your brain to be programmed to immediately spark your resistance.

Form Positive Habits

I hope that, by this point, I've convinced you that it's absolutely critical that you train mentally as well as physically. Most people train their bodies in the form of physical exercise a lot more than they train their minds. I can honestly say that I used to fall into that category. It's only now that I have the tools at my disposal to train my meta-physical world that I've realized the difference it makes.

The key is taking little, positive steps daily, which creates positive habits. It's important to live in the moment and not put too much pressure and stress on yourself by demanding giant leaps where little steps will mean long-lasting change.

I love the people who tell me they don't have the time; they are too busy, they wish they could but can't right now – maybe down the road. Sound familiar? Trust me, I've heard it all over the past eighteen years.

We all have the same twenty-four hours in a day. It's what we choose to do with those twenty-four hours that will make the difference when it comes to where we get with our journey. At the end of the day, that's what makes us all different.

You have the ability to choose where you want to be in life – it's your life. Most choose the path of least resistance and being comfortable. Instead, try getting *un*comfortable!

Do you have time for TV, movies, the news, the Internet, texting or talking on your phone? Think about all the things you make time for in your day without thinking about it. These are habits that you have engraved in your mind over many days, months and years. Facebook, anyone?

When it comes to the habits you create, whether negative or positive, they are formed the same way. When we are moving forward with a positive or negative habit, there is not a lot of difference in behavior. In the beginning, there's not much of an effect from either.

For example, if you work out once, it's not going to get you fit – just sore, right? Going to KFC one time isn't going to make you fat, correct?

But after about three weeks or so, you start to see a substantial change happening. You are building a neural pathway in your brain for whatever activity you are doing, whether it's mental, physical or spiritual. The first time is naturally the hardest with any new activity, but it's a heck of a lot easier after a few weeks.

Let's take me, for example. I started to take ice-cold showers, probably a year and a half ago, for the mental and physical benefits. In the beginning, my mind would tell me not to do it, and before I even got in the cold water, I would be shivering. It was tough, but I kept doing it anyway. I kept telling my mind to "shut up" and I would get in. Now, I can't stand hot showers. I actually enjoy the cold. I feel so much better afterwards. I'm more relaxed and my sleep is amazing. Imagine if I had listened to my logical brain telling me not to do it – I would be in the same place as I was eighteen months ago. You have to get uncomfortable to move forward in life.

It usually takes about thirty days to develop a new habit. This means you can make a new habit every thirty days, which creates twelve new habits in a year, which can change your life because your behavior has now changed. Who you become over the span of twelve months is now the new you.

By this point your identity has changed! And this is what you need to happen. This is what reprogramming your mind is all about. Without changing your identity, you will never change anything in your life.

So, with all this in mind, here are some ways you can take small steps each day to form some positive habits in terms of personal safety.

POSITIVE HABITS

- Every day, when you are driving your car or walking down the street, choose a vehicle and memorize its license plate for later recall.

- Each day, in different environments – whether your home, your office, a supermarket or a parking lot – make a point of noting the exits and fastest escape routes. Observe where any windows and doors are located, and the position of any obstacles between you and the exit. Repeat this a few times with each environment in order to build mental blueprints.

- Pick one person that you see each day, at work, on the bus or out the window at home, and categorize their appearance. Start with a couple of details, then, once you get into the habit, add more and more details to the list. See what you can remember about them later, and train yourself to recall more details.

■ When you're walking to and from your car, train yourself not to look at your cell phone at all, even if you receive a message. If you usually program your GPS on your way to the car, wait until you're inside the car with the doors locked.

■ Begin parking your car by backing it into parking spots rather than driving straight in, and cultivate the habit of always parking this way around.

■ Get into the habit of never visiting an ATM late at night. Each day, ask yourself whether you need cash for the evening and get your money out during your lunch break or when meeting friends during the day.

■ Stop using earphones when you are in public, whether on a walk, run or commute, and instead make a point to listen to what's going on around you. Each day, learn one new thing about your immediate environment or people in your vicinity that you would not have been aware of had you had earphones in.

■ Every time you take an elevator, take a moment to study who is entering it with you, and position yourself as close to the buttons as possible.

■ Each day, make a point to check the gas level in your car. Get in the habit of never letting it fall below half full.

■ Each time you go onto social media, assess your online behavior. Do you often check into places or post pictures of yourself at different locations, even when you're alone? Stop this habit. Before you post anything at night, ask yourself whether you are making yourself easy for a stalker and potential attacker to locate.

A lot of these habits will help you increase your awareness and alertness, which is integral to the next principle. And, again, they all begin with the mind. The first secret to stopping doing something is questioning yourself and realizing you are doing it. Each day, consciously assess how you behave and decide how you want to behave. That's when you can begin to cease one behavior and cultivate another.

Summary

When we think back to Sarah's story at the beginning of this part of the book, we can look at what happened to her and think about what could have been different if she had believed she was capable of escaping, if she hadn't frozen in fear, if she had tapped into her reason to prevail. In the next two parts of the book, we'll look at the things we can do to avoid being attacked and to escape an attack, but I want you always to remember that successful self-protection starts with what's going on in your mind. The first key is preparation.

In this part of the book, we've looked at the concepts of:

- Being selfish

- Taking responsibility

- Reprogramming your mind

- Defeating limiting beliefs

- Practicing visualization

- Adopting positive affirmations

- Fear as an alarm and fear as fuel

- Your reason to prevail

- Cultivating new habits

Make sure you've been through the exercises before you move on to the next part of the book, and then, let's go!

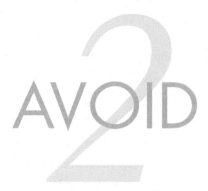

AVOID

*Using your instincts and intelligence correctly,
you may be able to avoid danger before it even comes close.
This is the ultimate goal in self-protection.'*

TONY TORRES

Jen was a schoolmate of mine who went backpacking before we went to college. She was tall, athletic and social, and she had her itinerary planned out, meeting and traveling with friends in different countries, while also doing her share of solo adventuring. She had successfully and safely traveled for months before she ran into trouble in Thailand. She didn't even realize how much trouble she was in until far too late.

A friendly couple ended up beside her on a crowded street that was swimming with tourists and market stalls, and they said hello. This was normal enough; being blonde and very fair skinned, Jen got a fair amount of attention when she was out and about in Asian countries. What happened next was a mixture of the usual and the surprising. They asked her about herself and where she was from. When they found out where she was going to university, they exclaimed at the fact that their daughter was going overseas to attend university in the States as well. They talked about their daughter and what she had in common with Jen. And then it struck them how brilliant it would be for their daughter to get a chance to chat with an American the same age before going over there to live and study.

They didn't overdo it. Jen thought it was a little strange they would want to take her to their home, but they'd approached her in a crowded place in a social way, the course of the conversation had gone naturally, and she didn't see the harm in spending some time with another girl, whose transition to overseas study she might make easier and less daunting. It's easy when you're travelling to meet and make friends with other foreigners, but more rare and precious sometimes to foster relationships with locals. She went with the couple to meet their daughter.

This is known in the industry as being taken to a secondary location. And it is something to be avoided at all costs. Jen was abducted and taken back to a house where a gambling ring was set up. She was stripped of her possessions, but made to take part in the games with what cash she had on her. When the money ran out, she was taken to an ATM and forced to withdraw money. When the limit was hit for cash withdrawals, she was taken to a jewelry store and forced to purchase gold on her credit cards until they were maxed out. Thousands of dollars. Only when she was bled dry was she released. But she is very aware she might not have been. Having been threatened and coerced for hours, once free, she was convinced she was being followed. She flew home as soon as could be arranged and with less than nothing.

I'm not telling you these stories so that we can pick holes in people's choices. You never really know how you're going to react in a terrifying situation until you are in one yourself. That's why, if an instructor or coach ever tells you in detail what you should do in a certain situation, you should find another instructor or coach. No one has the answer for what the exact response should be when it comes to an exact moment in time – there are way too many variables. That's why, when someone asks me what to do, I tell them, "It depends." You can only – and that's what this book is about – put yourself in a position to be as prepared as possible.

Logic dictated many of Jen's moves. Rational thinking – again, looking for the logical rather than acting on the obvious – has a nasty way of overriding common sense at times like this. If Jen had known the secondary location rule, and treated it as gospel, even if she didn't think she were at risk, she could have said she'd be delighted to meet the couple's daughter at a coffee shop, or at the market, and arranged a rendezvous in a public place. But once she was in their power and in their private sphere, that was it. She acquiesced to their demands, not knowing where she was except alone in a foreign country. And perhaps that did, in the end, save her life. She let her captors move her from location to location. Not knowing if anyone would understand her or help if they did, she did not make a scene on the way to the jewelry store or when they got there. The chance to avoid the experience had already gone – that was at the beginning, when this friendly couple were using charm and misdirection to distract her so that they could get what they wanted.

In this part of the book, we're going to look into some of the ways to avoid this kind of manipulation. Avoiding attack altogether is the best-case scenario, and this can be done through being alert and de-selecting yourself. Sometimes, listening to your intuition can make all the difference in the world, so we'll address what this looks like as well.

Weigh Up Your Attacker

Let's start by discussing your attacker. Who are you trying to avoid? What do they want? What don't they want? When, where and how will they attack you?

It's quite simple who your attacker is: an attacker is anyone who has intent to harm you or your family, emotionally, psychologically or physically. It could be a co-worker, a family member, a friend, a date, a boyfriend or the neighbor next door. It usually isn't the big, scary guy we all fear in our minds. It could be someone who makes us want to be friends with them, or it could be someone who looks like they need our help.

Attackers have one focus, and that is you. To be honest, they have a winner's mentality. They know what they want and will do everything in their power to get it. They think they can control you; they think they can intimidate you; they think they can manipulate you; they think you are weak; they think you are vulnerable; they think you will give up and give in to them. Their belief system is strong, and it fuels their actions. To be honest, this is the type of belief system that you need to adapt to conquer your attacker. You have to steal a page out of their book and use it against them.

What attackers don't prepare for is a victim who doesn't want to be a victim. What this means is that they don't have a plan B; they don't plan for the person who fights back, who doesn't give up, who causes them harm, who causes them to take a long time, who causes a commotion.

Attackers are looking for the easiest way possible to get their job done and get what they want from you.

You need to be able to recognize a threat, avoid your attacker and escape at all costs. You have to listen to your personal security system, which is your intuition. You have to think about what is at stake. Is it your life, your family, your future, your body or your property?

I will go over what to look out for and what behaviors to be aware of in the coming sections, but make note: Look out for strangeness, not necessarily strangers.

Look out for people who try to charm you, who disregard the word "No," who ask you a million personal questions, who want to know your schedule, who try to distract you. If something inside of you suggests that something is odd about this person, then listen to that voice and do the opposite of what logic tells you. Logic might tell you that they're just interested in you, that they're perhaps a little socially inept, that there's a reasonable explanation for them wanting something from you. Logic might tell you that you should feel flattered, to take it as a compliment, but beware your rational mind telling you how you should feel. Listen to your gut.

A TEDx talk worth watching is Apollo Robbins' The Art of Misdirection. He talks about how he's done research picking pockets to prove his point, and he has someone up on stage to show the audience what he's capable of. He notes the difference between attention and awareness, telling us you can actually attend to something without being aware of it. He talks about how attention steers perception, and he shows how it's possible to steer someone's attention and control their actions to your own ends.

While you don't want to live your life thinking that anyone being friendly is a master manipulator and a marauding attacker, it's also perfectly legitimate to put rules in place to protect yourself and be present to the possibility of danger. It's about being present, not being paranoid. Just as you wouldn't sit in a car doing ninety on the freeway without a seatbelt on, you can make it a rule never to agree to head to a secondary location with someone whose intentions you're not sure about, whether you think you know them or not.

What Do They Want?

To help avoid becoming a victim you have to be educated on what an attacker wants. Usually, it consists of one or more of the following three things:

1 **Your Possessions**

This could be anything that has value, such as your watch, jewelry, cell phone, tablet, iPad, iPod, wallet, cash, keys, and more. Anything the attacker can use or sell. This *is* the category where you can more likely avoid certain predators by not having items on display in certain situations, times and locations, which makes you appear to be an easy mark.

Your opportunistic thief is the one you haven't noticed in the bar, who wasn't originally out to rob you, but saw you leave your cell phone on the table when you went to the bathroom, pull out a wad of cash at the bar to pay for a drink before putting it back in your wallet, and exit the bar alone late at night. You leave the bar with your critical focus on the phone in your hands on the way to the bus stop, and you aren't aware that you're being followed. This is also the category where you can most likely avoid physical harm, or further physical harm if you've been sucker punched (taken completely by surprised), if you hand over what is demanded of you. It is not worth getting into a physical fight where you could lose your life for the sake of a valuable item.

2 Your Body

Wanting your body could mean a couple of things. The attacker could want to hurt you in order to take your valuables or so that they can bring you to a secondary location. They could also intend to do physical harm by sexually assaulting you.

In the latter case, this is not like the first instance where they only want your possessions, where submitting will mean you will likely not come to physical harm. Rape is physical harm, which also causes deep, damaging emotional and psychological trauma beyond physical injury.

Athena and Phil Thompson, authors of the book *Every Woman's Guide to Being Safe ... for Life,* talk about the dangerous, factually inaccurate myth that you shouldn't fight back or you'll only make your attacker more angry. The hundreds of rape survivors they have worked with have said that if they were in the same situation again, they would fight back viciously. They quote a survey of 1.5 million rape cases over ten years carried out by the American Justice Department, which reported that the injuries sustained by women who fought their attacker were no worse than those sustained by those who did not resist. Resistance did not increase the likelihood of further injury or death, and, most importantly, women who fought back more than doubled their chances of escape. Psychological recovery has also been shown to be quicker in those who fought, whether or not the attacker managed to perpetrate the rape.

3 **Your Life**

Your attacker might have the ultimate aim of killing you. This might be because they've sexually and/or physically assaulted you and don't want to get caught, or it might be that they're simply a psychopath and/or serial killer and this is just what they want to do. There is absolutely no reasoning with the latter – they do not play by the same social rules as the rest of us.

Identifying what an attacker wants can help to get you thinking when caught by surprise in an attack. The worst thing that can happen is that you freeze when you are attacked. Freezing means you have no options.

Remember, you always have options. Knowing ahead of time what an attacker wants helps load the dice in your favor. You need to get thinking as fast as possible and out of a state of denial.

Usually an attacker will do the following:

1 **Stalk you without you knowing,** waiting for the perfect opportunity, when they consider you are most vulnerable.

2 **Make contact with you in one way or another.**

3 **Attack you at the worst moment for you** – his best moment.

If they just want your valuables, great. Hand them over. Usually, an attacker will quickly leave. If they don't, then you can prepare for the fact that they want one or both of the other two things mentioned above, and you can take the appropriate action.

What don't they want?

An attacker doesn't want the following:

1 To Get Injured

Prey behavior induces predator activity. This is a big reason why attackers attempt to choose people they perceive to be weak, both physically and mentally. How many people do you think will attack a person who is alert to their surroundings, looks confident and is strong both mentally and physically? Not many, trust me! An attacker doesn't start their day by psyching themselves up to take on a stronger opponent who is confident and alert to what they are about to do. They want the person who is oblivious to the world, the victim who freezes, the prey who is apathetic and in denial. If they get a feeling that they may get injured before or during an attack, they probably won't choose you.

2 To Get Caught

Bottom line, an attacker doesn't want to get arrested. Their biggest fears are others seeing them and subduing them or the police getting there to arrest them right away. There is a reason why you should always try to be around people, places or things that will help prevent an attack. If the attacker senses they are likely to be caught, they will more than likely give up or not attack you at all. Just another reason not to be walking alone late at night in an isolated area.

3 To Have Attention Drawn to Them

This point feeds into the first two points. If attention is drawn to your attacker, they are more likely to be caught or hurt by someone coming to your aid.

When, Where and How?

We live in a relatively safe environment, contrary to the picture the media portrays. Though I've talked about the disturbing statistics, I'm not telling you to walk down the street as though there's someone behind every bush or around every corner waiting to pounce on you. I'm just talking about being alert to your environment and being present so that you can recognize a threat if one is there. If you don't want to be a statistic or end up on the nightly news, then listen to your intuition and use common sense.

Take a moment to think about what you are doing and whether it is a good idea or not. Taking the time to assess your situation and the choice you are about to make could help you avoid an attack.

Your attacker has the initial advantage over you for a few reasons, especially if the attack comes when you least expect it:

1. **They choose the time of day.** This is usually at night, but realistically could be any time of the day.

2. **They choose the place.** This could be anywhere, but it's usually where the attacker has privacy and the least chance of being caught.

3. **They choose the type of attack.** More than likely, they will take you by surprise, especially if you lack alertness.

4. **They have the intent.** Your attacker has the advantage in that they know in advance what they want from you.

5. **Their sole focus is on one thing only – you!**

When it comes to real violence, there are no rules. This is not a competition sport where two opponents have preparation time, training, consent and guidelines.

You must always be in a state of alertness about where you are, what time of day it is and whom you are with. You have to be alert for the people, places and things that could cause you harm as well as the people, places and things that can help you if needed.

This is all about stacking the deck in your favor. If you don't look like an easy target, and you don't put yourself in shady situations at shady times, you are less likely to get attacked.

But let me make one thing about my beliefs clear. Absolutely nobody deserves to get attacked. No one deserves to be hurt. Did Brock Turner's victim deserve to get raped behind a dumpster because she went to a party and drank like everybody else? No. Did Sarah deserve to get assaulted because she went into an office alone at the end of a Christmas party? No. Did Jen deserve to get abducted and robbed because she got talked into getting into a car? No.

The perpetration of violence and people taking advantage of people are sad facts about our world. The very need for a system of self-protection is a sad fact in itself. Perhaps you were almost someone's victim, and you don't even know that you evaded them. Or perhaps you actually have been someone's victim, which is terrible, and I'm so sorry for what you've been through. Or perhaps you've never come close to confronting violence and never will. Regardless, while I hope you never need them, I'm here to provide some tools to increase your chances of survival if the worst happens. I want to help you change your probability of experiencing violence by changing the way you think about self-protection and then changing the way you act. I want to help you understand and show you that it's so easy for things to go wrong, which is why we need to be vigilant.

Trust Your Intuition

Threat recognition is about identifying things that could potentially cause harm to you physically or mentally. This could be a change in a spouse's behavior or even a change in yourself, such as your intuition putting you on the alert.

You may be familiar with the idea of "a woman's intuition." Women are considered to have better intuition than men, but, in reality, this is only because it is triggered much more often. The simple fact is that a woman's intuition kicks in more frequently because they are more likely to have to deal with the potential of a date going bad, a relationship becoming abusive, sexual assault or violence at their place of work.

That nagging feeling in your stomach, that voice that keeps telling you something isn't right – these are signs that mean a threat has been recognized and you should take the appropriate action. Most of the time, if you can spot a potential problem ahead of time then you can avoid it and escape.

Your intuition is your body's own personal security system, and has been hardwired into you through thousands of years of evolution. It is part of your subconscious, and I can't tell you how it works in terms of the triggering of glands and hormones in the same way I talked about fear and the biological fight or flight response. It is just something that knows without knowing how.

Intuition can be seen as non-rational, a concept in the realm of feeling rather than thinking. The psychologist Carl Jung defined it as "perception via the unconscious," and neuroscientific literature sees it as sitting predominantly in the non-dominant hemisphere of the brain. The conscious and unconscious minds are often likened to an iceberg, with the conscious mind being the part sitting above the water, dealing with our conscious awareness and rational decisions, and the unconscious mind sitting below the water – the larger mass. This is where our unconscious beliefs reside, along with our memories, stored experiences and knowledge. And this is the part of us that guides our intuition.

You owe it to yourself to listen to that internal voice. It tells us when something is just not right. It talks to us by sending us feelings to experience, often in our gut, including nagging sensations of doubt, uncertainty, hesitation, suspicion and, most powerful of all, fear.

How often does something happen and we think to ourselves, "I knew something wasn't right." But because it was *just a feeling*, we ignored it. This is the problem with listening to our intuition, and the reason we don't tend to – we don't get a bulletin telling us we were right. We don't get concrete evidence. That's what I meant when I said you may be someone who has actually avoided an attack without knowing about it, either before or after. Perhaps you unconsciously felt something and took a course of action based on that feeling that may have saved your life, but you don't even remember doing it because you didn't get the bulletin.

We shouldn't ignore our gut feelings and talk ourselves into ignoring them. Sometimes we do find out that we were right, and our bad feelings are substantiated, but by then it's too late. This happened at a high school in my state. One of the teachers turned out to be a pedophile. He was only discovered because another teacher – the head teacher in fact – came under investigation. People couldn't believe it. Except that they *could* – it turned out kids had said things, parents had felt things, but folks had been too polite to put up a hand and make any noise about it. Maybe it was the bystander effect all over again, with no one wanting to take responsibility in case they were wrong, assuming that if they were right, someone else would've said something by now. But it turned out the rumors, the bad feelings, *were* right.

People had taken on board the limiting belief that there was no way a respected *teacher*, having gotten to a position of authority and served in it for so many years, could be taking advantage of the kids, and they'd rationalized and explained away the indicators. In the case of both teachers, more than one person came forward afterwards, saying, "I knew something wasn't right." They had known without "knowing," without being able to substantiate the feeling with hard evidence. Yet, if enough people had raised a question, putting forward some of the indicators and kids' comments as cause for concern – all of which had been dismissed on an individual basis – then the answers and the evidence would have come to light much sooner.

At the end of the day, if you get that feeling that something just isn't right, it probably isn't. You need to learn to trust yourself.

Intuition Drills

Being so subjective, it's difficult to see how you might be able to develop your intuition, and you won't see the results in the same way as you would if you were working on your fitness, for example, but it is possible.

Meditation, mindfulness, creative activities such as drawing and writing, and dream journaling are all things which have been shown to help develop your intuition. If you feel like you're a bit out of touch with that aspect of yourself, it is worth exploring further.

Here are a couple of simple drills for you to try. The first is focused internally; the second is focused externally. There are no right or wrong answers, and you'll find that the frustration with talking about and developing your intuition – as well as the barrier to listening to it – is the inability to confirm your observations in a concrete way (as previously discussed}. But the important thing is to concentrate and tap into your inner feelings. This is how we access our inner wisdom.

Drill #1: Intuition Drill—Introspection

Do this drill at home and make sure that you are in a relaxed state, alone and free from any distractions. I am going to get you to ask yourself a series of reflective questions in order to dig deep and get in touch with your intuition.

Ask yourself the following, slowly and in a relaxed manner, and give the answers that come up for you. You can start by giving a general answer, but then try to be more specific, especially when considering why you've given a particular answer.

- What do you consider happiness to be?

- Why?

- What makes you happy?

- Why?

- What behavior do you display when you're happy?

- How do you react to things?

- Why?

- What do you consider anger to be?

- Why?

- What makes you angry?

- Why?

- What behavior do you display when you're angry?

- How do you react to things when you're angry?

- Why?

- What do you consider fear to be?

- Why?

- What are your fears?

- Why?

- What behavior do you display when you're afraid?

- How do you react to things when you're afraid?

- Why?

If you had difficulty answering any of the questions, ask them again in a different way. And if you only gave a short answer, ask yourself the same question again. Repeat the question until you go deeper and are able to find the answer within yourself. After all, in this internally focused drill, the questions are about you, so you *know* the answers.

If it helps to write things down, then do this exercise with a pad and paper. That said, don't edit any of your answers (this can be a particular temptation if you do this on a computer). Expand on your answers by all means, but add detail rather than changing anything. Your first, gut response is your intuitive response to the question.

I want you to do this drill alone rather than with a conversation partner in order to articulate the answers without any filter whatsoever. When someone asks us a question, we often have our gut answer, but then think before speaking, engaging that rational part of the mind. Sometimes we'll say what we were *going* to say, but other times we filter or alter our answer depending on our audience, or due to our own self-judgment, sometimes without even being aware of it. Part of the aim of this exercise is about breaking the habit of concern about what another person will think about your words or actions.

This is particularly important in situations where your personal safety is at stake. The fear of being perceived as rude has gotten women hurt, raped and killed, and their attacker has played on that fear, using it to override objections and causing the victim to shut down the voice in their head and heart telling them something is wrong. If someone is being genuine toward you and you are rude to them, the worst thing likely to happen is their being offended. They might decide not to like you very much, they may communicate that dislike to you and to others, and they may even get angry. However, in contrast, the consequences of *not* being rude to someone who intends to cause you harm can be deadly. If your gut says get out of an interaction, then get out. There are cues to be alert for, which we'll look at in the next section, but your best course of action is to follow your gut impulse and not worry about trying to rationalize it.

Drill #2: Intuition Drill – External Focus

This drill is going to ask you to tap into your inner feelings, but this time with an external focus. Take the following steps in a public place; for example, in the store if you've gone out to do the shopping.

- Quickly scan the people around you, making brief eye contact.

- Really observe who is around you and what they are doing as you walk down the aisles. What are they doing with their hands? Are they holding a basket, pushing a trolley, or just grabbing a couple of items quickly by hand? What items are they picking up? Are they checking their phone?

- Pick one person. Without staring, what is their body language telling you?

- How do you feel about them?

- What do you imagine they are thinking?

- How do you imagine they are feeling?

- Pick other people from around you and ask the same questions of yourself.

- As you glance around, do you get the impression that anyone is worried about something? Happy about something? Late for something? Hungry? Are they going home to a family or meeting a partner or do you feel like they live alone?

- Look for a couple shopping together. How do they interact with one another? What do you think their relationship is like? How do they make you feel?

- Watch someone for a moment. What does your gut tell you about them?

This time, while I've asked you to articulate your perceptions, I haven't burdened you with asking yourself *why* you feel a certain way – why, in this context, doesn't matter. What matters is letting yourself feel whatever feeling comes up for you, observing the feeling that has come up, and articulating what that feeling is, even if it's not very clear.

Again, you're asking and giving yourselves the answers, so you're allowed to be completely honest with yourself.

Yes, some of these questions are invasive. Some of your perceptions may be spot on and you'll never know. Some of your perceptions may be off the bat and you'll never know. Some of your perceptions may even be insulting to the people you're observing. But this is between you and your intuition – it's between you and you. Something is giving you a signal and that's leading to your feeling. You just don't necessarily know what the signal is. Imagine you pass a couple and you get the feeling that they're in an abusive relationship. You don't know why. Later, if you actually found out it *was* an abusive relationship (and, trust me, you walk past couples like this all the time), you might turn around and think, "I knew there was something," and with deeper thought about it (rather than immediate denial about how you're probably mistaken), you might even pin down the signs and signals *why* you got that feeling in the first place.

One rule in this drill: you're allowed to be rude – you're only speaking to yourself. And you're allowed to feel the way you want. Not only that, but if you ever feel uneasy, suspicious or scared, even if you don't know the reason why, you're allowed to act on those feelings and remove yourself from the situation, even at the cost of being rude, even at the cost of being insulting. This is about you giving yourself permission to listen to your intuition.

I want you to be more alert to *strangeness,* not necessarily *strangers,* in your day-to-day life, so also ask yourself these questions when you're in a situation with people you know, not only in an environment where you don't know the people around you.

Try this in your office, for example. Regardless of how your co-workers are acting, your answers may be colored by what you know is going on in their lives or your previous experience with them. Of course, throughout the course of our interactions with others, all of these questions may very well run through our heads at lightning speed, in our subconscious, and we're making snap perceptions without being aware of it. Think of a time you've heard someone's gone home because they're sick or they've suffered a loss, and you've said or just thought to yourself, "I thought they weren't looking well," or "I had a feeling that something was off with them." You may not have known till the moment that you articulated it that you *had* observed that thought or feeling. What I'm asking you to do here is practice bringing those feelings to the fore, and consciously answer questions that might highlight them to you.

Meanwhile, when we're in a public place, we're not necessarily looking for signs of danger or pegging people as serial killers; we're allowed to feel positive feelings here, as always. And we're allowed to access a spectrum, as always – not only "I feel good," or "I feel bad." In a high-risk situation, the warning bells may well be a little stronger than when you're asking yourself to identify your feelings here, and that's because your body is trying to communicate with you. What we're trying to do is broaden that channel of communication so you don't instantly dismiss it.

Be Alert

In order to pick up on the signs that may trigger your intuition, it helps to be alert. People rarely look at alertness as a critical part of personal safety, but it is one of the most important. Alertness isn't awareness, which is passive. You can be aware while you're asleep, for example, and wake up when you hear an unfamiliar noise. Alertness, on the other hand, is active. You're in the moment.

As Tony Torres says, "Being alert, or in a state of alertness, prepared to respond to danger or emergency, is ultimately more important than just being aware of your surroundings. Being merely aware without an emergency response plan, strategy or doctrine simply means that you may see danger coming but not be able to avoid it."

Alertness is so vital, even *during* an attack. When the attack is going on, it helps to broaden your focus and make mental notes on your attacker, so when you escape, you can help the police with an accurate description to aid them to capture and arrest the individual.

But alertness is most key when it comes to being able to avoid attack altogether.

What is it to be alert? It means you're being present; not sleeping awake! It begins with the distinction I mentioned before – concentrating on having broad vision and extended external focus rather than narrow vision and critical focus trained on some distraction, such as a cell phone, iPod or book.

But what are we being alert for? If we're alert, then as well as being aware of elements of our surroundings when it comes to the people around us and the environment we are in, we can also learn to look out for certain warning signs in our interactions. Our intuition may already be tingling, but knowing indicators to look out for can confirm or enhance your feelings in an instant.

In *The Gift of Fear*, Gavin de Becker calls these "survival signals," and describes them using the following terms:

■ Forced Teaming

This is where someone manipulates you by establishing common ground in order to strike up rapport. The idea is offered up that you're in the same predicament together, and that you've struck up a partnership, even if you haven't agreed to it. An indicator of this is the use of the words "we" or "us." They might barrel through your objections, establishing you on the same team, making it seem rude if you continue to refuse their offer of assistance, for example. The appropriate action is to mentally, verbally and physically refuse to acknowledge the partnership. Deny it, refute what they say, keep saying "No," and keep your independence rather than being swept along.

■ Charm and Niceness

These might sound like positive traits, but if someone is trying to charm you with intent, or they're being nice to you in order to manipulate you, then it's a tactic you're going to want to see through. As de Becker says, 'niceness does not equal goodness' – it can be a control-seeking strategy, a way to make you trust where trust is not warranted. The appropriate questions to ask yourself are whether someone is trying to charm you and why they might be trying to control you, and see what your gut says in response.

■ Too Many Details

This is a way to establish whether someone is likely to be lying to you. Adding excessive details to a statement can be a ploy to make a lie seem more credible. You may not be questioning their veracity, but the liar knows they aren't telling the truth, so they add unnecessary embellishments. The appropriate thing to do is to question the context of the encounter – the details and lies are all there to distract you from what your attacker really wants. If someone is working hard to establish rapport and feeding you details, consciously look to the simple context – nothing they say will change the fact that they are a stranger attempting to gain entry into your home, for example, or that you have asked them to leave several times and they are still accosting you. Don't fail to see the wood for the trees.

■ Typecasting

This is offering some form of insult in order to get you to bite, and get you to stay and engage with the attacker to prove them wrong. It might be suggesting you look too snobbish to talk to them, which will prompt you to talk to them so you aren't labeled a snob. The appropriate action is to ignore such comments – the verbal response, and attempting to prove them wrong, is exactly what the attacker wants. Maybe they're not an attacker, but just someone in a bar who has studied pick-up routines and is offering you a "neg" (a form of backhanded compliment) in order to get you to engage with them. The "neg" makes you feel unworthy so you feel you have to prove your worth to them. Even if the intent isn't sinister, it's worth seeing it for what it is – a manipulation device.

■ Loan Sharking

This is where you're offered unsolicited assistance in order to put you in an attacker's debt. It is where someone will pick up and start carrying your groceries without asking, or they'll buy you a drink even if you politely refuse and say they're just trying to be nice. And maybe they are a genuine gentleman just trying to be nice, but it doesn't stop the action being a sign of the more predatory behavior out there – or stop the fact that it evokes a feeling of being put under an obligation. When worried about being rude, the appropriate action is to be rude anyway. Remember that you did not ask for help (and if you did need help, you'd be much safer choosing someone to ask, rather than having someone choose you because you look like you need help), and that it can be a form of exploitation.

■   The Unsolicited Promise

When you don't ask for a promise and get one regardless ("I promise I'm not a serial killer," "I promise I won't hurt you,"), then it is cause for concern. Such promises are made by an attacker to persuade you of their good intentions, yet they offer no guarantee; the promise is only there to convince you to trust them. The appropriate response is to be suspicious, and the question to ask yourself is, "Why are they promising me this?" It's likely because they see your doubt about their intentions. And that very realization can reflect your own doubt back at you so you can take heed of it.

■   Discounting the Word "No"

Someone ignoring your saying, "No" is easy to spot. If you think to yourself, "Maybe they don't think I mean it," then it's time to make yourself crystal clear. If you say, "No," but then let someone carry on with what they're doing, they'll perceive that they've changed your "No" into a "Yes." You don't want your attacker to perceive that they've even got a "Maybe." It gives them what they want – control. If they refuse to accept rejection – whatever they are asking for or offering – then it is a massive sign to get away from them. The question to ask yourself is why they won't take no for an answer. The appropriate action is never to give in, or let it become a matter for negotiation or conversation. Make it very clear that "No" means "No," and, as de Becker says, 'remember that "no" is a complete sentence.'

Alertness Drills

I'm going to take you through some alertness drills now, which will illustrate exactly the kind of behavior you can practice to increase your level of alertness. The intuition drills were about looking inward (even with an external focus); these alertness drills are specifically about training your powers of observation and conscious awareness.

Drill #3: Alertness Drill - SLLS

This is a drill to practice every morning. It helps you build situational awareness and become alert to your surroundings. It's an army drill I learned from Retired Lt. Col Scott Mann, an ex Green Beret who spent eighteen years in Special Forces and twenty-three in the U.S. Army.

1 Stop:

- Each morning, find a quiet spot outside.
- Crouch down and take the soil or rocks into your fingers.
- Allow yourself to slip into the role of predator.

2 Look:

- Scan your horizon from left to right, then right to left, slowly. Take it all in the way a big cat surveys the landscape from a tree branch.

3 Listen:

- Close your eyes.
- Listen for the most distant sound.
- Picture it in your mind as if you are floating above it.
- Listen for the closest sound.

4 Smell:

- Take in every smell that you can.
- What belongs?
- What doesn't?

Drill #4: Alertness Drill – Driving

Every single time you're in your car, you're making high-risk predictions regarding what the other drivers on the road are going to do, and taking the appropriate action to keep yourself safe. Often, you'll say after the event, "I knew they were going to pull out in front of me," or before the event, "I bet they're going to cut me off." But reading the road, with seconds to make critical judgments that keep you safe, you may not know how you know these things. You've seen the signs so quickly you don't even know you've seen them, and you listen to what your inner driver tells you to do.

On the road, you often rely on your intuition to protect yourself, without even realizing you're doing so, because there's no time to think about it. And while you generally play by the rules and hope others will do the same (slow down if you're merging in front of them, do not overtake on the wrong side, do not run a red light when you're turning at the junction, stop if you're stopping in front of them), you have to be alert all the time for those people who you know don't play by the rules (will speed, will have their critical focus on their cell phone, will drive drunk, will have a child on their lap). Practicing alertness while driving is, I hope, a given, part of being able to qualify for a license at all, but perhaps it's a skill that becomes so familiar that we come to take it for granted, and we don't necessarily think about it – like looking both ways before we cross the road. It's habit.

This drill is about bringing your level of alertness to the fore, not so much assessing it (though that's good, too) as becoming consciously aware of it.

This is what principle-based self-protection is all about. It's about letting the instincts that have been engraved in us over thousands of years take over. It's about not complicating things and disrupting what our bodies want to do. If I whip a ball at your face, you instinctively react by covering (protecting your head/face) or by pushing away the danger. By contrast, technique-driven systems disrupt/interrupt what your body wants to do, causing a huge problem.

So, next time you take a drive (and you can do this as a passenger – "backseat driving" – as well as a driver), do the following.

- Talk out loud, constantly, every single turn of the wheel.

- Describe what you see – signs, the color of things, the environment you're in, etc. Describe every single action you take and why.

- Describe the other cars on the road in your periphery – not just their appearance, but your perception of their driver's behavior.

- What do you predict they are going to do?

- Do they do it?

- How did you know?

- Repeat, repeat, repeat.

Drill #5: Alertness Drill – Profiling

As we talked about in the section on intuition, we're constantly going about our days filing snap perceptions in our brain about the people around us and about our environment. We may not even be aware of these perceptions unless we're triggered to think about them, and when we are, we may not be able to quickly trace them back to the signs and signals that caused our perception in the first place. This drill, again, is about raising our powers of observation, and bringing to the fore our ability to be consciously aware of our unconscious perceptions.

The next time you have an uncomfortable feeling, maybe you won't waste valuable time explaining it away (looking for the logical rather than acting on the obvious), but assess the environment for the cause of the feeling. If it really is nothing (i.e. something non-harmful that your body has unknowingly picked up on as a threat), then your brain will learn, and not raise that alarm again. But *something* has caused the feeling, even if you're not aware of it.

This is about increasing our alertness so we become more aware in general. Some people, including detectives and magicians, are considered to be uncannily perceptive, with otherworldly powers of deduction. They can amaze a roomful of people, like the fictional Sherlock Holmes or the very real Derren Brown, despite and sometimes because of the detailed explanations they give for their mental leaps. However, their perception isn't uncanny, and their powers aren't otherworldly. They have simply honed their skills through sharpening their powers of observation and alertness. They may have done this to such an extent that it appears remarkable, but it is very much in the realm of the possible.

This is something to practice whenever you're out and about. The more you repeat this exercise, the more you'll find your powers of observation improve.

- When you next leave your home, regardless of where you're going, notice every single person you come across.

- Don't just practice this drill when it comes to strangers and dismiss the acquaintances and friends you come across in the course of the exercise. Look at everyone.

- You can consciously observe them for a second without staring or making them uncomfortable. It's amazing what the eye can pick up and process in a millisecond, so a whole couple of seconds can provide plenty of material.

- Make a mental note of some feature of each person, whether it's something different from everyone else or something they have in common with others.

- After each person passes out of your line of sight, can you recall what they were wearing? Their expression? The action they were taking?

- Several hours later, try to remember specific people whom you passed and observed. Which are easiest to recall and why?

Drill #6: Alertness Drill – Mental Blueprinting

Mental blueprinting sounds technical, but, in essence, it is very simple. It is about forming that path of least resistance in your mind ahead of time, so that it's there in your mental files when you need it. This is why we practice fire and shooter drills in offices and in schools. While performing the steps physically can enhance the experience, it can also be effectively done through intense visualization, as we discussed in the first part of the book. This increases your level of alertness in an emergency because you have a plan. You could even call it cheating.

Initially perform this exercise in a relaxed state, preferably alone, without any distractions.

- Pick a place you visit frequently, such as a local restaurant, your workplace, the grocery store, your usual parking spot, even your own home.

- Picture it in your mind. Picture it vividly. Call up the emotions that you usually feel when you are in this location, and really *feel* them. You are *never* feeling nothing, even though that might be your first thought. Take some time and tap into your usual state of mind.

- Now look around you. If you are having trouble with this, then physically go to the location and perform a run-through. You can even take pictures on your phone to look at later.

- Visualize this scenario: You are in this location, in a particular spot in this location. You need to escape.

- Where are the exits? Visualize them exactly.

- What is the best escape route? Envision yourself taking it, one step at a time.

- The best escape route is blocked. Which is the next best escape route? Envision yourself taking it, one step at a time. Feel the emotions coursing through you.

- You need a weapon. Picture any improvised weapons available in your location. What are they? Where are they? Envision yourself grabbing your improvised weapon, one step at a time.

- Your weapon of choice isn't available. What is the next best thing? Where is it? Envision yourself grabbing it, one step at a time.

- Visualize your escape, holding your weapon. You have gotten away. What positive emotions are you feeling? Relief? Triumph? Are you looking forward to letting your loved ones know you are safe?

- Now, return to your favored escape route. Describe it to yourself aloud, relaying the details of the visualization. Include a description of the improvised weapon and the plan B for both the secondary route and the secondary weapon if your first choices aren't available.

- You can also talk through this escape blueprint with a partner. Have them ask you a question, for example: "You wake up in bed in your home in the middle of the night. You need to get out immediately, grabbing an improvised weapon on the way. What do you do?" Describe the route to them in detail. The most important aspect of this visualization, as with any that you practice, is to assign it a positive outcome associated with positive emotions. Do not imagine you fail or consider what that would look and feel like. Do not let that be a defeatist pathway that you've called to existence in your brain.

Why are we doing this? If it's a simple route to the door, as it's likely to be in your home, why bother? Why not just ask the question, "How would you leave your house?" and then answer it simply in a line? Why are we doing it in a relaxed state when we are calm and can think straight?

Because in a scenario where you need to use this blueprint, you will not be in a relaxed state. True stress inoculation is very difficult to achieve, and you are going to be highly stressed. You don't even know exactly how stressed. You will be unable to replicate the exact level of stress of escaping a burning building, for example, without setting the building on fire and then attempting to escape it. You won't truly be able to imagine what it's like to dial 911 in the course of a brutal assault unless you pick a fight, goad someone into beating you, and attempt to use your fingers to hit the right buttons while the blows are hailing down on you. Here, we're trying to achieve the opposite of the saying "familiarity breeds contempt." We want to go over a scenario so many times that it is ingrained in us. We've thought about it once, twice, a hundred times – and now when we need it, our brain is going to offer it up immediately.

Try this. Turn on every sound-playing device in the house. Blare them full volume. Every radio, every TV, every laptop, every phone with a speaker. Turn on the tumble dryer if you have one. Turn on the shower or taps if they're noisy. Make the alarm on the stove sound. If you have kids, get them to scream, shout, jump around upstairs, bang things and make loud noises. If you have a partner, get them to yell at you – insults, nonsense, incomprehensible noises, anything. Now recite whichever escape route you've been trying to visualize in detail.

This scenario doesn't even approach the battery on your senses and the pressure on performance you will experience in an emergency situation. Do what you can in advance so you don't go blank when it really matters.

Go over things in your mind until they are just there, embedded in your brain. Until you can answer the question without thinking, like when someone asks you to count to ten when you're engrossed with something else or there is a major distraction at play.

Practicing the above drills will mean that you become more alert. Being more alert is its own reward, but it will also mean that you'll show the signs of being alert to your potential attacker without even thinking about it, and this is what can make the difference when it comes to de-selecting yourself from attack.

De-Select Yourself

De-selecting yourself is about telling your attacker that you are present and aware. We've talked about *them* sending you signals that you can pick up on; this is about *you* sending some signals of your own. Confident body language and an air of alertness will reduce the probability of your being seen as an easy target, and this may well be the difference between getting attacked and being left alone.

Remember, prey behavior will induce predator activity. Think for a moment about a how a lion walks around compared to a gazelle. Which one has a commanding presence and which one doesn't?

A lion naturally has their head held high and chest out. Their presence is commanding wherever they go. A gazelle, on the other hand, often has their head down, raising it when they sense danger, but in a twitchy, unconvincing way.

What is an attacker looking for: a lion or a gazelle?

An attacker wants a "soft" target. A soft target is someone who is not paying attention to their surroundings and lacks situational awareness. An attacker wants the easiest target they can find because they are lazy; they don't want someone who is difficult and takes a lot of energy and effort to overcome.

If you are daydreaming or distracted, talking on a cell phone, texting, playing on a tablet, listening to music or reading a book, you're often oblivious to what's going on in the environment around you. However, it's your powers of observation that can keep you safe from harm, so you really need to exercise them. As with anything, the more you practice them, the better they become.

To help you understand the difference between a hard and soft target, here is a table comparing the qualities and actions of the two:

SOFT TARGET	HARD TARGET
They walk slowly.	They walk briskly.
Their head is down.	Their head is up.
Their shoulders are slouched.	Their shoulders are back.
Their critical focus is on the device in their hands.	Their vision is broad and external – they scan the environment and make brief eye contact with people around them.
They have an air of distraction.	They have an air of alertness
Under the impression they are being followed, they will sneak a furtive look over their shoulder or in a mirror for a threat.	Under the impression they are being followed, they will turn square on and assess their environment for a threat.
They exhibit timidity.	They exhibit self-confidence.

Being a hard target makes you a less desirable victim for a would-be attacker. Attackers have one goal in mind: to go the path of least resistance. If an attacker perceives that you are too much of an effort, or that you come with higher risks of them getting hurt, getting caught or drawing attention to themselves, they will move on to easier prey.

If an attacker thinks that you are going to be a problem, chances are they won't select you. Remember, they don't have a Plan B, so they want to make sure Plan A works. Don't let them consider you, and you automatically don't let them implement their plan with you as their prey.

But how exactly do you walk with genuine confidence? Confidence comes from having knowledge about personal safety. Understanding and practicing the mental and physical tools you'll find here will help you become a hard target, someone who knows and believes they have it in them to prevail against violence. Knowing in yourself that you are more aware, more alert, and have the tools at your disposal that can keep you safe, will translate into the way you carry yourself – your very bearing.

If you don't want to become a victim of violence, start by being alert, not only when it comes to your surroundings, and people, places and things, but also when it comes to how others perceive you. This is the key to de-selection.

De-Selection Drills

Here are a few drills you can practice with the aim of cementing your awareness of the elements of de-selection and increasing your ability to actually put them into practice.

Drill #7: De-Selection Drill – Attacker Frame of Mind

This is one to practice after rereading the section on weighing up your attacker. Remember what they want; remember what they don't want; remember what they're in control of; remember how they select their target.

Choose an occasion when you're out and about in public and do the following.

- Put yourself in an attacker frame of mind.

- Regardless of where you are, notice every single person you come across.

- Don't practice this drill just with strangers and dismiss the acquaintances and friends you come across in the course of the exercise. Look at everyone.

- Assess each person who crosses your path as though you are a predator looking for prey. Decide what you're after (their possessions?) and study your potential victim. What is their body language saying? Where is their critical focus? Who is making brief eye contact with people, with you? Who projects an air of confidence? Who seems distracted and completely oblivious to everything and everyone around them? Who looks like they would struggle and cause a scene and potential injury to you, and who looks like it would be easy to get what you want from them?

- As you move on, you can let your intuition do the assessment without consciously and painstakingly running through the checklist. Make a snap decision. Is this next person a hard target or a soft target? If you were an attacker, who would you pick?

- Later on, recall the details of the people you came across in the course of this exercise. Which people most easily spring to mind and why?

Drill #8: De-Selection Drill – Movie Analysis

The next time you watch a movie or TV show and there's an element of violence (as there so often is), I want you to take a series of steps while you're watching to analyze what's happening. Don't just play armchair quarterback and judge the actions of the characters involved. The reality is that your actions in a violent situation will depend on a number of variables. What I want you to do is relate what you're watching to the principles you're learning so that you can train yourself to see your options.

- Watch a violent attack scene.

- Analyze the lead-up to the violent scene from the perspective of the victim (rewind if you can). How did they act?

What were the consequences? Did they make themselves a soft target? How?

■ Identify pre-attack clues from the attacker, such as stalking, making contact, body language, their breathing, their expression. Did they exhibit any of the survival signals we ran through earlier, such as putting the victim in their debt or disregarding the word "No"? Were there signs that the victim missed that an attack was coming?

■ Analyze the lead-up to the violent scene from the perspective of the attacker (rewind if you can). Enter into that attacker state of mind again for this part. What did they see? Why did they choose this victim? How did they act?

■ Who prevails in this violent encounter and why?

Drill #9: De-Selection Drill – Subtle Eye Contact

These next couple of drills step away from analysis and put you in the driver's seat. Knowing what you now know, what can you do to make yourself a hard target and de-select yourself from attack? These aren't drills I want you to practice once or twice; these are drills I want to become a part of who you are and how you act on a daily basis.

The first drill is about making eye contact with other people when you're out in public.

■ Attempt to make brief eye contact with people around you. There is no need to be intense about this and stare at someone until they look at you. Naturally glance at them. Through the course of these drills, you should be getting into the habit of glancing at everyone. If your gazes meet, good. If not, never mind, but maybe try them again at another juncture if you're sitting on a bus together, for example, rather than passing each other in the street. Perhaps the reason they don't see you is that their critical focus is entirely absorbed with something else, which is fine, and an observation you've now made. You are just doing this to let people around you know that you are there and that you are present.

- How do you feel when you make eye contact with some-one in this way? If you are naturally extremely shy, and it makes you feel something just short of nauseated, then work on this. How? Visualization and attaching a positive emotion to eye contact. This emotion could be a feeling of confidence, of empowerment. You know who is around you – you have met their gaze. You have noted the color of their eyes, the expression on their face, simply by hav-ing glanced at it. Do you have a limiting belief that meet-ing someone's gaze is challenging or rude or forward? You need to discard this belief and replace it with a new one. Meeting people's eyes lets them know you are there. It lets them know you are alert to your environment and to them. It lets attackers know you are a hard target.

Drill #10: De-Selection Drill – Walking with Confidence

This drill is about how you carry yourself when you walk. Is it really that important how you walk? Yes. Remember, an attacker chooses you.

- Every single time you walk from A to B, keep your head up. This is the only way to meet people's eyes as per the last drill. At the risk of repeating myself, your critical focus should not be on a smart device, book, music, or other distraction.

- Place your shoulders back and your chest out. These do not have to be exaggerated movements that make you look like you've puffed yourself up. These are movements that basi-cally mean you are *not* slouching. You have good posture.

■ Scan the area around you. This means you have broad rather than narrow vision, and your external focus is extended. Notice things about your surroundings. The very fact you are making mental notes and are conscious of your level of alertness will increase your air of confidence.

■ How do you feel when you walk around in this way? Do you usually walk this way, only now you're hyper conscious of it? Or is it different from normal? Does it make you feel uncomfortable? Then you need to work on this. Practice it physically but also visualize it mentally when you're in a relaxed state. Again, you need to attach a positive emotion to it. This emotion is confidence or empowerment. You know what is going on around you – you have noticed things about your surroundings, simply by keeping your head up and your vision broad. Do you have a limiting belief that people who walk this way are arrogant or cocky or think themselves above other people? You need to discard this belief and replace it with a new one. Walking confidently lets other people know that you are strong. It gives you presence. Seeing you scan your surroundings lets them know you are alert to your environment. It lets attackers know you are a hard target.

Summary

This part of the book has been all about the best-case scenario – avoiding attack altogether. Hindsight is nowhere near as valuable as foresight, so why do we tend to lament at one, ascribing it worth, and scoff at the other, ascribing it none? Listening to your intuition, that inner voice that wants to keep you safe, isn't acting paranoid; it's being present to your body's security system. Your unconscious perceptions move faster than your conscious thoughts, and your rational mind will look for the logical rather than act on the obvious.

Looking at all the stories and examples, why wouldn't you act on your gut feeling? If it's for the sake of not seeming rude, then I hope I've gone some way toward proving that the consequences of being rude are relatively mild in comparison to the worst-case scenario. What Jen, from our opening story, and other survivors of attack have in common is that they are willing to see what they could have done differently. They are aware of a lack when it came to their level of alertness. Day to day, are you aware of any lack in yours? Are you willing to do things differently?

In this part of the book, we've looked at:

- What your attacker wants

- What your attacker doesn't want

- When, where and how you may be attacked

- Trusting your intuition

- Increasing your alertness

- Recognizing survival signals

- Being a hard or soft target

- De-Selecting yourself

In the next and final part of the book, we'll look at how to escape when you haven't been able to avoid a violent encounter and have no choice but to engage.

ESC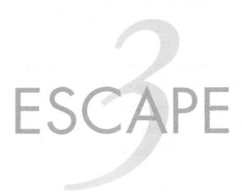APE

*'Your only goal if you are placed in a violent situation
that you could not avoid is simple; to escape.'*

ATHENA & PHIL THOMPSON

L ily was a nanny who came to me because her mother insisted she look
into self-protection after hearing a horror story about a woman in the
same line of work. She was one among the minority of clients who
hadn't experienced violence before, so she said she found it hard, initially, to tap into the emotions during visualization exercises. She was a naturally
confident and self-assured young woman, but while her primary reason for
training was to give some comfort to her mother, she still applied herself
100 per cent to understanding the concepts and practicing the principles. She
admitted to having a variety of misconceptions about the nature of violence
and the idea of self-protection, like a lot of people. Unlike a lot of people,
she worked wholeheartedly to turn them around. A couple of years later, she
got in touch with me to tell me what had happened to her, and to thank me
for giving her the tools to escape being another horror story.

Lily had been working for a man, looking after his two young children on
various occasions over several weeks. She described him as nice. Normal.
He was in finance. He'd checked her references and been friendly without
feeling too friendly and encroaching on her personal space. He was polite

and considerate, and tipped her generously on the occasions he engaged her services. He was separated from his wife, so he didn't have the children all the time. When he did, the main reason he would hire her was for the occasions when he'd have to be at the office late, or if he had a dinner meeting that he couldn't reschedule. She said he was warm and loving with his children on the occasions she saw them together.

One night he came home late from a dinner meeting. He had messaged her during the evening, as usual, to confirm the likely time he would be home, but had also messaged her a little later saying things were running longer than he'd thought. When he got home, she opened the door to him. She immediately perceived he was incredibly drunk.

He grabbed her forearm when she let him in and immediately entered into an angry diatribe against his ex-wife. His focus quickly switched to her, comparing her favorably to his wife and saying Lily would never do what his wife had done to him. He stumbled forward and kissed her on the cheek. Hyper alert, Lily silenced the voice that rose up saying she shouldn't be worried because his kids were asleep in the house and he had always seemed like a nice guy. She immediately engaged her brain and decided that what she needed to focus on was being careful to do nothing to escalate the interaction, and taking the appropriate action to get away. She shifted her stance into one where using physical tools would be easy for her, but which displayed non-violent body language to him. From her feeling about the situation, and the fact that he was currently blocking the exit, she did not immediately employ physical force in order to escape the house.

She didn't wrest her arm away from him, didn't tell him to calm down, didn't threaten him and didn't raise her voice. He carried on talking, getting increasingly worked up. When he took a breath, she lightly touched his hand where it gripped her arm, made a sympathetic sound and asked him calmly whether he wanted a drink. This disrupted his flow and distracted him. He released her arm, likely prompted by her non-threatening touch reminding him of the grip he had on it. She took a step back and repeated the question. He said yes and she went ahead of him into the kitchen. She asked him if he wanted to sit down at the counter, which he did, and then prepared them each a drink, implying she would sit with him to have it, chatting the whole time she did so, telling him about the games she'd played with the kids earlier in the evening. Thrown off base, he didn't say much in return.

After setting the drinks down on the counter, she took a sip from hers, then casually said she just needed to grab her phone from the other room. She walked back through the living room, picked up her bag and headed for the exit. Opening the door, she calmly called over her shoulder that she hadn't realized the time and had to go, and briskly left. Lily told me that she was glad she had listened to her intuition, which had told her that the situation could escalate unpleasantly if she didn't change the course of things and get away. She also said she was glad she'd gone through our self-protection training, which meant she quickly assessed her options and followed a strategy, rather than having a knee-jerk reaction. She said the man later got in touch with her and apologized for his behavior, but she decided to avoid ever being in a similar situation with him and left his employment.

I'm going to go on to explain defuse and de-escalate tactics in more detail. I'll talk about when they're appropriate (and when they might not be), and provide some exercises to help you practice them. These are the verbal and physical engagement tools you can use to defuse and de-escalate a situation with the sole purpose of getting away and to safety. Where these fail, or are inappropriate, or you've been taken completely by surprise by someone who's intent on causing you physical harm, then you have to engage physically, and with immense force, immediately. This means striking first if you can, and with intent to do debilitating harm. The latter sections of this part of the book cover the precursors to physical violence and the tools and targets you need to be aware of to most effectively attack your attacker.

In any instance, the primary aim, where you haven't been able to avoid violence, is to escape it. Where you manage to incapacitate your attacker, there is no question of taking further violence in vengeance. The reason for teaching you how to hurt and injure someone in the most destructive and vicious way is so you can *get away* as quickly as possible. I originally considered calling this part of the book "Engage," because the tools here are the verbal and physical engagement strategies to use during a violent encounter. But they are not the end-goal. The ultimate aim is to *escape*. How you do so is through appropriate engagement. So let's look at how to engage your attacker.

Defuse and De-Escalate

Simply put, to defuse and de-escalate is to talk your way out of a situation between you and your attacker. If someone can talk, they can walk away.

Defusing or de-escalating a situation is a part of your strategy to lower a person's guard and keep their ego in check. It's important to trust your intuition here. There is no formula for knowing with any certainty when these tactics will or won't work. If you feel as though you're under threat and these tools aren't going to make any difference, then you need to look at your other options for appropriate action.

The important distinction here is that you have identified a specific danger and are taking a pro-active approach to make the situation less dangerous. This may include using speech and body language to attempt to calm an angry subject.

You can also use your limbs and your environment to create physical barriers that can slow down or impede an explosive attack.

How to Use Submissive Tactics

Acting in a submissive way when it comes to violence is a strategy in your de-escalate and defuse toolbox. This does not mean you are giving up and not resisting – it means that you are acting in a certain manner in order to effectively defuse certain situations, or, in some cases, in order to lower an attacker's guard and get close enough to strike.

These tactics ensure the attacker sees you as a victim. In this scenario, you appear extremely vulnerable and non-threatening, which is an essential part of your personal safety plan. This gives your attacker a false sense of security and enables you to attack your attacker without warning.

Being submissive is typically used in a situation where an attacker wants to rape or sexually assault you because the attacker needs these three things to be successful:

1. **Privacy**

2. **Control**

3. **Dominance**

To make them think that they have these things, you can employ submissive tactics to play the victim role. This means using words and behaviors, with congruous body language, that reinforce the perception that the attacker is in control. This lulls them into a false sense of security and lowers their guard, increasing your chances of a successful escape.

Appearing submissive consists of the following elements:

- Using a fearful voice, i.e. speaking in a shaky, quivering way.

- Reiterating to your attacker that they are in control and that you will do what they want.

- Keeping your vision broad. Don't look straight into your attacker's eyes. This can be perceived as a challenge, as well as meaning you may miss what their hands are doing, which is the real concern in this situation.

It is also good to act submissive when an attacker is using a weapon, because they are more likely to put down this tool of intimidation if you convince them they don't need it to maintain control.

How to Take a Passive Stance or Non-Violent Posture

The first thing to be aware of is that communication is roughly made up of: seventy per cent body language; twenty per cent tone of voice; ten per cent spoken words.

Being passive means that you maintain non-threatening and non-challenging communication while using congruous body language. You can't say one thing and have body language screaming the total opposite. Just yell a profanity at a friend or relative while leaning in for a hug and see how they react.

Appearing passive consists of the following elements:

- Using a non-threatening voice, speaking in calm but assertive tones.

- Having neutral body language, neither aggressive nor submissive; for example, neither leaning forward nor cowering.

- Being empathetic and getting the person to think; for example, by asking them a question. This lowers the pressure cooker.

There are many benefits to maintaining a passive stance or a non-violent posture. You don't want to get into a fighting stance, as they teach in martial arts or in some types of self-defense, because your body language will say that you want to fight, even if your words claim the opposite.

An attacker won't hear what you have to say; they are going to hone in on your body language.

Your passive stance is part of your personal safety plan. It is a psychological manipulation tool to lower your attacker's guard and increase their ego and confidence. You want your aggressor to feel like they are in control, that you are the perfect victim. In their mind, they are thinking that you won't fight back and cause them harm.

Put simply, you don't want an attacker who thinks you can fight back, otherwise they will be ready for you. Essentially, you want to attack them when they least expect it and effect a role reversal where they become the prey and you are the predator.

This is position one in the combative toolbox that I'll talk about later, but I'm going to describe it here as well – it's that important. So here are the elements of a passive stance or non-violent posture:

- Your hands are up in front of your body.

- Your palms are open.

- If standing, you have a bladed stance, which means one foot slightly in front of the other, standing slightly side-on to your attacker (this places your vital targets – your center line – out of their direct line of attack).

If your attacker does attack you, having your hands up in a passive stance will help maximize your reflexive response and protect you from their attack.

A passive stance will allow for pre-emptive striking because at close quarters, your hands are quicker than your attacker's eye can follow. You will be able to land any strike you want with your hands before they are able to react, which will enable you to cause the first injury, making it possible to cause other injuries with your strikes.

In addition, the passive, non-violent posture will allow you to gather critical intelligence, increasing your situational awareness of escape routes, multiple attackers, weapons, obstacles and improvised weapons.

It will create distance between you and your attacker as well as giving your attacker very limited ways to attack you.

How to Defuse a Violent Situation

When we are in a social setting and there is verbal communication, there is always the option of walking away and defusing the situation.

The key to de-escalating and defusing a situation is to avoid confrontation at all costs. Remember that you control the situation because you control how you respond. You control the most important person – you! And this gives you an opportunity to attempt to control the situation from your perspective. Use the following verbal and physical tools:

- Use a calm and assertive tone.

- Employ empathy by making a comment that shows you putting yourself in your attacker's shoes. This absorbs tension.

- Don't look into your attacker's eyes, as they may take this for aggression.

- Give your attacker a way out; make it sound like they are right.

- Never tell people to calm down, challenge them or threaten to do something to them.

- Never try to make it appear that they are doing something wrong.

- Interrupt your attacker's thoughts and distract them. A person can't really think about two things at once – they can only overlap. Distract your attacker verbally by asking a question or introducing some dialogue that will shift their focus away from their immediate goal. This gets your attacker thinking, and it gives you time to assess your surrounding environment, your attacker, and how they are responding.

- Physically distract them by grabbing something non-threatening, such as your wallet, to divert their attention/critical focus.

If the situation hasn't gotten physical yet, your attacker needs your help to get them to the next level. Don't allow it to happen.

Defuse and De-Escalate Drill

This drill is one to practice with a partner. It will help you practice the elements that we've run through above.

DRILL #11: DEFUSE AND DE-ESCALATE DRILL – ROLE-PLAY

Run through different scenarios with a partner. These could include road rage, where a driver has pulled over to confront you, or arguing with your spouse, a fellow employee or someone you do business with. Role-play a scenario with your partner.

Focus on defusing the situation by using the tools we've discussed. This is not to get physical. Train yourself to talk someone down, lowering the pressure cooker by using your body language and voice.

- Adopt a passive stance.

- Don't look into your attacker's eyes, as they may take this for aggression. Do not tell them to calm down, challenge them, threaten them or accuse them of wrongdoing.

- Use a calm and assertive tone and employ empathy by making a comment that shows you putting yourself in your attacker's shoes.

- Distract your attacker verbally by asking a question or introducing some dialogue that will shift their focus away from their immediate goal. Physically distract them by grabbing something non-threatening, such as your wallet, to divert their attention/critical focus.

- Give your attacker a way out; make it sound like they are right.

If your efforts to de-escalate or defuse fail, and the danger targets you and chooses to do harm, an engagement begins.

Precursors to Physical Attack

When an attacker decides to get physical with you to get what they want, you must use physical tools to prevail against them. But what are the signs and signals to look out for so you can attempt to pre-empt their attack?

The following table runs through the precursors to physical attack. Be alert and you'll know if the situation is about to escalate into a physical encounter.

VOCAL	FACE/EXPRESSION	PHYSICAL MOVEMENT
Their breathing becomes faster and more shallow.	They seem to stare at/look through you.	They shift their body weight and change their stance.
Their tone of voice changes.	Their skin tone becomes pale/white.	Their body tenses.
Their speech pattern becomes short and repetitive.	Their skin tone becomes red.	They make big, jerky movements, or gesture aggressively.
Their volume rises, their voice loud and aggressive.	They show more white around the eyes.	They suddenly become very still, their center of gravity low.
They suddenly become speechless after talking non-stop..	They glance around quickly as though to see who is around.	They lunge forward.

As well as observing the signals from your attacker, it is worth making note of the behavior of any other people who may be around. If others are moving away from the attacker fearfully, this will inform you that their bodies have picked up on a cue that anticipates physical violence.

Your Combative Toolbox

If you are sucker punched, meaning you're attacked by surprise, then you must get through the initial onslaught of the attack.

How do you survive an attack and then prevail against your attacker?

Simple – you let your instincts do their work. They will cause you to compress or extend parts of your body to protect your vital areas (brain, eyes, throat), so you can think, breathe and move. Then you can use your gross motor tools to attack your attacker.

This is a principle-driven approach (as opposed to the technique-driven approach of martial arts), so the first thing I'm going to do, before talking about the physical tools themselves, is take you through a set of principles to follow.

Principle #1: Use Gross Motor Tools, Not Fine Motor Skills

Gross motor skills are simply large actions using your hands, arms, legs, feet or your whole body, as opposed to the fine motor skills, which involve a complicated series of movements using more muscles. Gross motor tools work with your body's natural reactions, enhancing your body's natural ability. They don't require you to learn a certain technique. We're talking about simple, straightforward strikes – not a complicated combination of techniques that take years of practice to get right.

Principle #2: Use Closest Tool on Closest Target

This principle allows you to improvise and respond to your attacker using whatever tools are best available in the moment to disrupt their attack. We're going to run through the tools and targets below – this principle is about making things easy and effective for yourself under pressure. It's very simple to remember.

Principle #3: Use Soft Tools for Hard Targets and Hard Tools for Soft Targets

We're going to run through the different tools and targets below, and this principle is pretty self-explanatory. You'll be most effective when you use a soft tool on a hard target (e.g. your palm to the attacker's head), otherwise you're likely to break something. Similarly, you'll be most effective when you use a hard tool on a soft target (e.g. your fingers in the attacker's eyes), otherwise your strike won't have much impact.

Principle #4: Go for Primary Targets

The primary targets are the ones you're naturally protecting on your own body – the eyes, throat and head. This is where the real difference between street fighting and combat sports kicks in. Combat sports train consenting individuals, often of the same gender, weight class and skill level, who are prepared ahead of time, to engage on mats or rubber flooring in competition with one another. Most importantly, there are rules and regulations concerning targets and techniques that are considered unacceptable in the competition. In a real-life scenario, there are no such rules. There's a reason that attacking the primary targets is often prohibited in sport – they're the most effective places to cause debilitating harm to your attacker, resulting in serious injury. This is appropriate where you're in a situation where it's necessary to protect yourself from harm.

The key points to remember during an attack are to remain conscious and alert, stay standing if at all possible, and gain time to improve your level of consciousness. If you've been knocked down to the ground, return to an upright position.

If you have missed the attack precursors and been struck, your sole job is now to reverse the attack.

When you are attacked, it is because the attacker has seen you as prey. Reversal is, in essence, changing the predator/prey mentality by simultaneously protecting yourself and taking action to defeat your attacker.

Your goal is to derail and interrupt your attacker's intent by creating a physical and psychological imbalance and reversing your role from prey to predator. This is critical. You cannot control how your attacker reacts but you can control your own mindset.

To engage is to enter into battle. At this stage, we bring our physical tools to bear and apply disruptive force until we resolve the conflict.

There are a couple of strategies worth mentioning here before we get into the tools and targets.

Strategy #1: Strike High to Low or Low to High

This is causing a disruption to your attacker's physiology and psychology by messing with their senses. They are being attacked all over their body in no set pattern – it's a mental barrage.

Strategy #2: Lower Your Center of Gravity and Step Into Your Opponent

This will give you more force behind your strikes to help you incapacitate your attacker.

Strategy #3: Strike in Threes

Don't just strike once and be done. Strike repeatedly and inflict all the damage you can.

The important thing to do is disrupt your attacker's ability to move or apply force in your direction. Once this is achieved, you can escape and get help.

The key, and probably the most critical part of using your physical tools, is to go full throttle!

Below are the gross motor tools I recommend because they are the simplest and easiest to use during a high-stress attack. Remember, during an attack, anything on your body can be used as a tool to help damage, incapacitate and cause trauma to your attacker so you can escape.

Self-Protection Tools

NON-VIOLENT POSTURE/PASSIVE STANCE

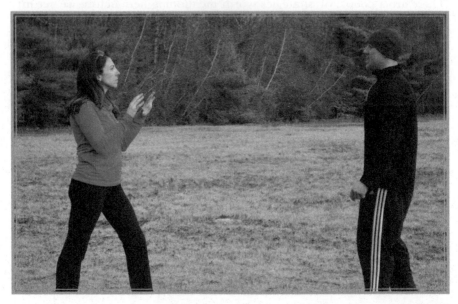

Passive Stance w/ Indignation

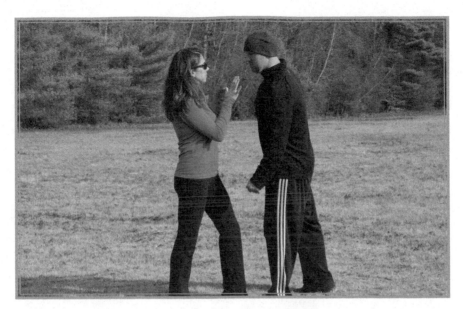

Passive Stance w/ Encroachment

This is used when protecting your personal space in close quarters. It can lower your attacker's guard by communicating passivity through body lan guage, help you scan the environment, and assist you to strike the attacker first by giving you the element of surprise. Most importantly, in close quarters, taking this stance means your hand can move quicker than your attacker's eye can follow. It can be used standing or from the ground, the important aspects being that it both protects your center line and increases your reflexive response. This means you can either extend or compress parts of your body to protect yourself when being attacked, and then engage your attacker. You're like a spider luring your prey into your web.

- Your hands are up in front of your body.

- Your palms are open.

- If standing, you have a bladed stance, which means one foot slightly in front of the other, standing slightly side-on to your attacker (this places your vital targets – your center line – out of their direct line of attack).

COMPRESSED PROTECTION

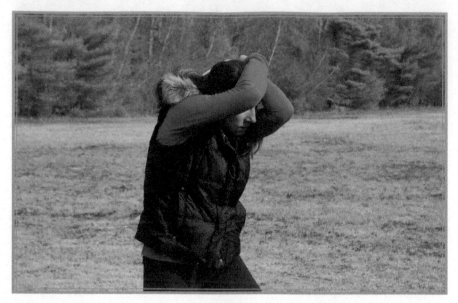

Compression Protection

Compression is what your body does reflexively to help protect your head against a strike from an attacker. It also enables you to effectively crash into your attacker. Compressing or covering is instinctively hardwired into us to protect us from harm. It's what your body wants to do before anything else.

- Place one arm over your head, in front of your face, grabbing the back of your head with one hand.

- With your other hand, grab your wrist. This position protects your head.

- To attack from this position, drive your elbow into the attacker's throat or sternum.

EXTENDED PROTECTION

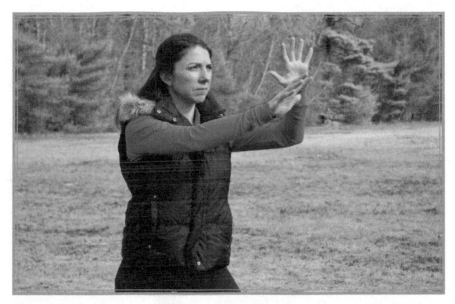

Extended Protection

Extending parts of your body helps to protect against a strike from an attacker. Extension is stronger than flexion when it comes to protecting yourself. An arm that is extended, for example, has more power when holding off an attacker than a flexed arm.

- Make sure your arm is outside ninety degrees, i.e. not flexed.

- Make sure your hand is splayed.

- Use the forearm bone of your arm like a hockey stick and drive it into your attacker's sternum and clavicle or neck, as if cross-checking.

Combative Tools

PALM STRIKE

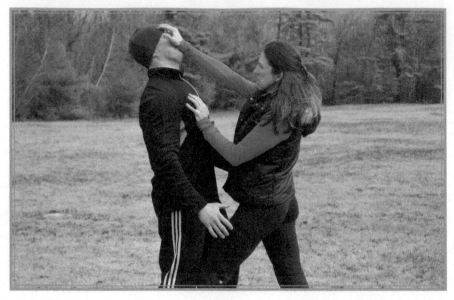

Palm Strike to the Face

This is used to strike the face or groin.

- Imagine palming a grapefruit or watching a basketball player palm a basketball. Don't aim for a small area.

- Use an open hand and aim for the whole face of your attacker when you strike.

- You can also turn your palm to face the sky and strike the groin area of your attacker. Imagine the motion of a bowler or softball pitcher – this is exactly how the arm will move to strike the groin. It helps to anchor onto the attacker with your other hand to give you more power.

HAMMER FIST

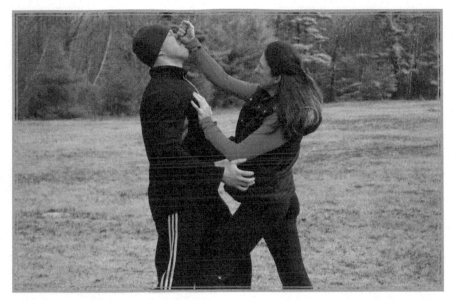

Hammer Fist to the Face

This is used to strike the face, head and body.

- ▦ Picture peddles on a bike and how they go around and around. Imagine holding onto the ends of the peddles while making a fist.

- ▦ Move your closed fist in a cycling motion and strike the attacker.

RAPID EYE BLITZ

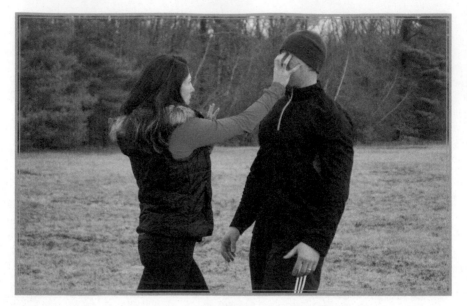

Rapid Eye Blitz

This is used to strike the attacker's eyes.

- Use an open hand.

- Slap the attacker's face in a downward motion.

- Rake your fingers into the attacker's eyes as they move down over the face.

- Repeat the move using your other hand.

- Use strikes from alternating hands in rapid succession.

SENSORY OVERLOAD: BLEND/RIP/TEAR

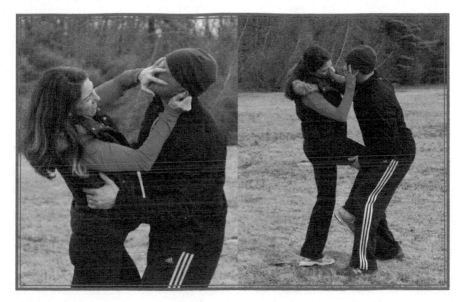

Sensory Overload (left); Sensory Overload with Knee Strike (right)

This is used in extreme close-quarter situations.

- Once you are in close quarters, imagine that your hands and fingers are like magnets and the attacker's face is like metal.

- Rip, tear, scratch and claw with your fingernails into the eyes, throat, ears, nose, etc.

- Resemble a cat, ripping apart the attacker's face.

- Keep moving – do not pause and become motionless at any point.

- Strike down low as well as ripping and tearing up high.

FOREARM STRIKE

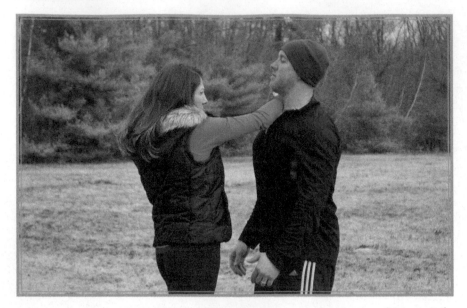

Forearm Strike

This is used to strike the face, neck and head. It is very effective from a passive stance – the beauty of this strike is that it can come from your non-violent posture so your attacker doesn't see it coming. It can cause a lot of damage.

- Use the bone in your arm as your weapon.

- Use the same motion as the palm strike. Picture cracking your attacker with a hockey stick across his face, in a cross-check motion.

- At the same time, use your forearm as an extended frame to create space.

SLAP

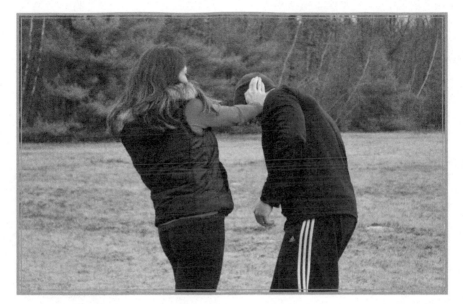

Slap

This is used to strike the side of the head and face.

- Use an open hand.

- Anchor with your opposite hand. Anchoring means grabbing and holding onto your attacker, using him as grounding to drive more power through your strike. This makes it more effective and causes more damage.

- Rotate your hips, use your foot as a pivot, and strike.

KNEE

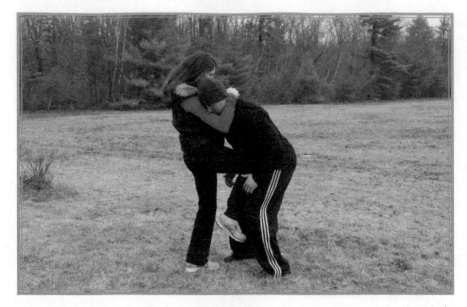

Knee Strike

This is used in close-quarter situations.

- Anchor your hands against your attacker. Hand placement can be anywhere – what you are doing is grounding yourself on your attacker to increase the power of your knee strike. Your knee will have a lot more power if you can hold onto your attacker by the head or upper body.

- Make sure to strike with the knee bone, not the thigh muscle.

- Use your knee to strike various parts of the body, especially the groin and face.

SHIN KICK

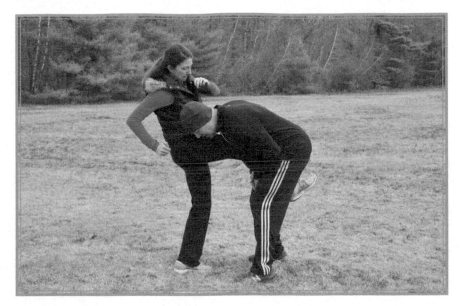

Shin Kick to Groin

This is used to strike the groin or side of leg. We use the shin because it will feel like being hit by a baseball bat as opposed to a small foot.

- Use your shin bone.

- Strike the groin in a swift, upward motion.

STOMP

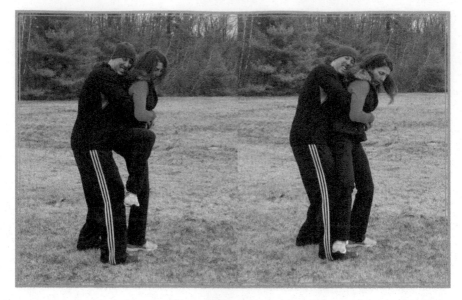

Foot Stomp

This is a good tool to use if grabbed from behind or in extreme close quarters, while standing.

- If being held from behind, use your heel to strike the top of your attacker's feet.

- If you have got your attacker to the ground, use your heel to crush their ribs and face when they are down.

ELBOW

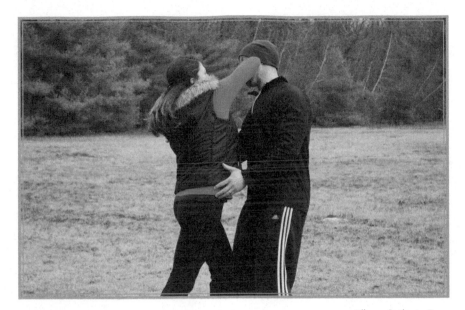

Elbow Strike to Face

This is used when in extreme close quarters.

- Use the bone of your elbow, not the muscle in the forearm.
- Thrust and strike the neck, face and head of your attacker.

SPIT

This can be used in extreme close quarters to provoke a flinch response. This creates an opportunity to attack your attacker.

- Aim at the face, the eyes in particular.
- Attack immediately afterwards.

BITE

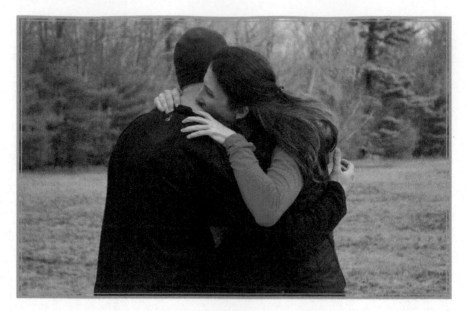

Biting Neck

This is used in extreme close-quarter situations. It helps create space in which to attack your attacker.

Bite the attacker anywhere on the body. There is no right or wrong way to bite or best place to bite. Whatever you can get to in the moment, going for the closest target to your mouth, is what you bite. What you are doing is both physically damaging and psychologically damaging to an attacker because of the savageness of the attack. You are causing a predator/prey switch. Make sure you growl to add to the experience. Trust me, it will work!

VOICE

Where possible (there may be occasions when people are literally scared speech-less), use your voice while you are attacking. Even if you are in a remote place and doubt anyone will hear, you are raising the idea of being heard and catching the attention of others in the attacker's mind, and it may work to distract them.

Pick Your Targets

Almost every part of the body is a target. You need to choose the targets that will cause as much damage (or as much distraction) as possible to the attacker, to allow you the opportunity to escape.

How you are grabbed or struck will have an impact on what is available to you in that moment. Your attacker may dictate your next move by decreasing your options, but it's important to go through the list in order to know what options are left open to you.

This is not an exhaustive list of targets, but below are the most important areas of the body to damage on an attacker.

PRIMARY TARGET: EYES

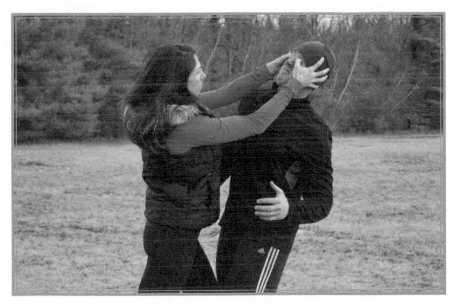

Eye Gouge with Thumbs

The eyes are a primary target. Regardless of a person's size or strength, it is very easy to cause damage to their eyes.

Here are a few ways to attack the eyes:

- Gouge, which means digging your finger deep inside an attacker's eye socket to rip his eye out.

- Tear/scratch, which means using your nails to tear/scratch the eyeball to disrupt his vision.

- Rake, meaning to rake/drag your fingers down his face to tear/scratch/rip flesh and do damage to his eyes along the way.

- Poke, meaning to push a finger into your attacker's eyes to disrupt vision.

- Spit, meaning to spit saliva to cause a flinch response. Even faking this is effective – fake spitting into someone's face and see the response you get.

- Throw or spray something in them, depending on the circumstance; it could be sand or dirt, chemicals, hot sauce or pepper.

PRIMARY TARGET: THROAT

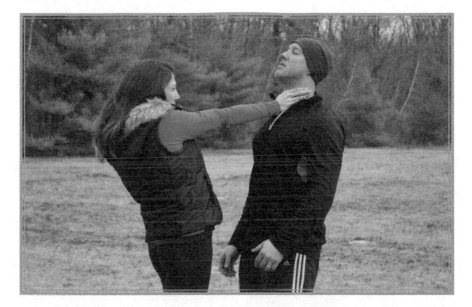

Throat Strike with Web of Hand

The throat is another primary target. It takes very little force to attack the throat and cause extreme discomfort, a coughing/choking fit, or worse.

You can choke or strangle your attacker by shutting down the blood supply or oxygen to the brain.

Make sure you are in a life-or-death situation before striking the throat because damaging it can cause extreme injury and even death.

Here are a few ways to attack the throat:

- Hammer your fist into the attacker's windpipe.

- Strike your elbow or forearm into their trachea. Use your elbow (in the same motion as reaching around to put on a seatbelt) to strike the attacker's neck/throat/face.

- Crush their trachea with your fingers.

- Palm strike.

- Web of hand strike to the trachea. The web of the hand lies between your thumb and index finger.

- Choke or strangle the attacker's neck.

PRIMARY TARGET: HEAD

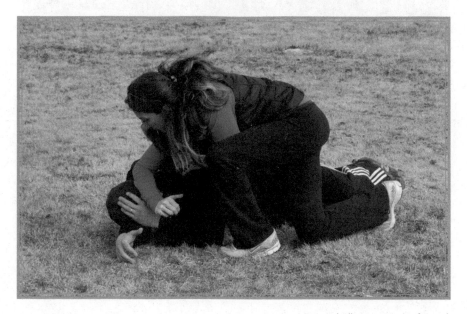

Ground Elbow to Back of Head

Striking the eyes and throat first disables your attacker's ability to see and breathe; however, the head is still a primary target when it comes to shutting down an attacker.

Countless videos on YouTube, highlight reels from combat sports, and real-life experience all tell us that the head is an extremely hard target. However, it can be damaged to shut down an attacker.

Here are a couple of ways to attack the head:

- Use your open hand to strike the side or back of the head. Do not use a closed fist because you might break your hand.

- Use a horizontal, vertical or diagonal elbow to strike the front, side or back of the head.

EARS

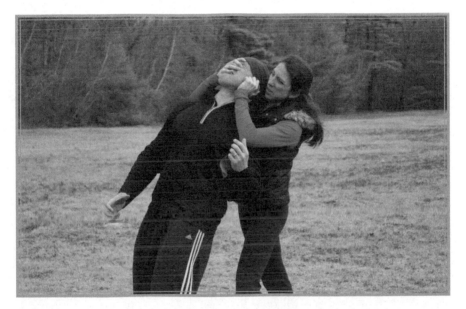

Sensory Overload with Ear Ripping

Ears are good to strike as they are a sensitive area and can throw off someone's equilibrium, especially if you burst their eardrum. Bursting someone's eardrum causes a lot of pain, and damaging the ear will distract the attacker, offering you more targets or the opportunity to escape.

Here are a few ways to attack the ears:

- Slap with a cupped, open hand to make sure pressure from the slap directly impacts the eardrum.

- Use an ear as an anchor by grabbing it with one hand and striking with the opposite hand.

- Grab/rip the ear. The attacker's reaction to this will give you other targets to exploit.

- Tear the ear off altogether. This will cause psychological as well as physical impact.

NOSE

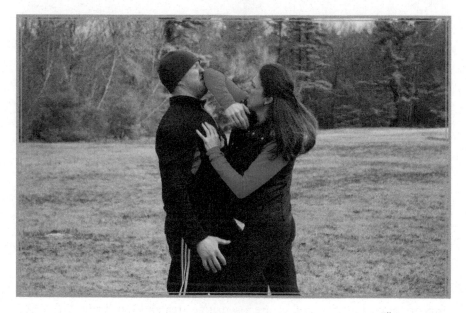

Elbow to Nose

Striking or crushing the nose causes a lot of pain and it also often causes the person's eyes to water, creating further distraction. The nose can also be used to manipulate the head position of an attacker.

Here are a few ways to attack the nose:

- Hammer your fist or elbow into the attacker's nose.

- Aim for the whole face, but palm strike the nose.

- Get your fingers up the nostrils of the attacker. Use your fingers to rip the nasal cavities, and hook your fingers to control the movement of the head.

- Head-butt backwards into nose/face if the attacker is behind you.

GROIN

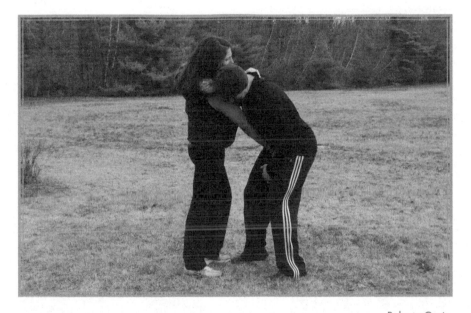

Palm to Groin

The testicles are a great target as they can cause debilitating pain. Damaging these creates great distraction.

However, please don't solely rely on a groin strike to subdue an attacker. In a high-stress situation, an attacker might not feel pain in the usual way. In most cases, it will just slow them down, giving you opportunities to attack other areas to shut them down for good so you can escape.

Here are a few ways to attack the groin:

- Hammer fist strike up into the attacker's groin.

- Grab and crush the testicles.

- Knee the groin.

- Shin-kick the groin area. This will be like getting crushed by a baseball bat.

HAIR

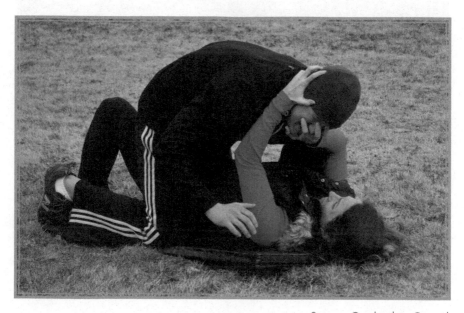

Sensory Overload on Ground

If your attacker has hair, use it as a target to help you escape. Going for the hair will give you an opportunity to attack other areas.

Here are a few ways to attack the hair:

- Grab it and use it as an anchor to control your attacker's head.

- Pull.

- Rip.

FINGERS, KNEES AND TOES

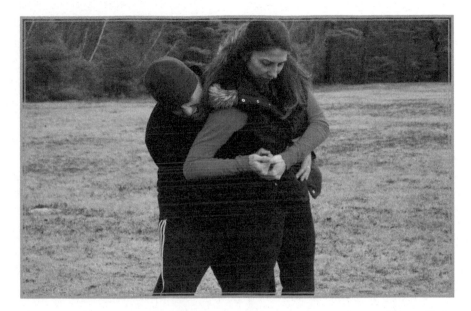

Palm to Groin

Any of these joints can be manipulated to cause damage. Here are a few ways to attack the fingers, knees or toes:

- Kick the knee.

- Drive your shoulder into the knee.

- Break or snap the fingers by grabbing them and bending them.

- Stomp on the foot and toes to break them.

Escape Drills

Now I've taken you through these physical tools, I want you to go through a couple of drills that will help you cement the moves in your mind so you can call upon them if you ever need to, which I hope you never do.

DRILL #12: ESCAPE DRILL – MOVIE ANALYSIS

I want you to go back and look at a violent scene in a TV show or movie again. If you want, look at the same one you did before and analyze it from this new perspective. The more you look at, the more you will benefit.

- Watch a violent attack scene.

- Analyze the lead-up to the violent scene from the perspective of the victim (rewind if you can). How did they act? What were the consequences? Did they throw fuel on the fire? How?

- Identify pre-attack clues from the attacker, such their body language, their breathing, their expression. Did they exhibit any of the precursors to physical attack?

- Put yourself in the place of the victim. Does it look like there was an opportunity to verbally defuse the situation before the attack or would this have been pointless? How would you have acted in their stead? How do you think you should act in the context the victim found themselves in?

- Analyze the physical tools that the victim uses when fighting their attacker. Are they using gross motor tools or attempting to use fine motor skills/techniques? Can you identify opportunities they missed to incapacitate their attacker? How would you have acted physically in their stead? How do you think you should act in the context the victim found themselves in?

- Who prevails in this violent encounter and why?

DRILL #13: ESCAPE DRILL – ATTACK VISUALIZATION

This visualization drill is the same one I went through in the first part of the book when we talked about it as a performance enhancing technique. The difference this time is the level of detail you'll be able to add to the visualization, using the verbal and physical tools we've been through in this later part of the book.

1. **Create an environment.** (Picture yourself after work in a parking lot, or walking to your car after shopping. You could be out on a first date.)

2. **Create a frame of mind.** (You're exhausted from a long day, stressed out, or distracted.)

3. **Think of a potential situation.** (Someone wants to ambush you to steal your valuables or rape you.)

4. **Develop the scenario.** (You are walking to your car; a guy comes up to you and alarms go off in your gut. Or you're back at your date's apartment and he's pressuring you to stay. There are a number of scenarios you could go through here.)

5. **Create a confrontation.** (Picture getting attacked. Imagine how you would move.)

6. **Slow it down.** (Observe the strikes and reactions from your attacker.)

7. **Create a response.** (See yourself attacking the attacker.)

8. **Create an outcome.** (Enact how you overcome your attacker and escape.)

The most important aspect of this visualization, as with any that you practice, is to assign it a positive outcome associated with positive emotions, as we discussed earlier.

Rely On Your Mind

Coming up to the end of the book, let's dial it back a moment. We've been through a lot of different aspects of self-protection in this part of the book, and learnt a lot of stuff, but I want you to know that the most important lesson is to keep things simple and straightforward.

When a situation arises such as a confrontation or violent attack, there are three integral things that you need to do:

1. **Breathe** – Exhaling will lower your heart rate and help you to relax. When a confrontation arises or a surprise violent attack occurs, your heart rate will go through the roof. Exhaling will help bring it back down quickly and breathing steadily will improve the oxygen flow to your brain.

2. **Think** – Thinking keeps us from freezing. You always have options. If you aren't thinking and acting, you are freezing and losing. Weigh up your options and tap into your emotions.

3. **Move** – Get moving as fast as you can; this will help your mind to move as well. Take the appropriate action to escape the danger and keep yourself safe.

Preparation increases confidence, which translates into a positive mental attitude, enhancing your chances for success. Preparing yourself and believing in yourself helps load the dice in your favor, giving you a mental edge over your opponent, and by going through this book and its exercises, you've taken a step to prepare yourself to face violence.

Many of you may have heard from one person or another that they consider themselves safe because they carry a gun or pepper spray in their purse.

You may also have heard from instructors, friends, family and the news that people are safe because of their cell phone or some other device they have on them.

They are all wrong. These things are a false comfort generating a false feeling of security. The truth of the matter is that you can't rely on anything other than yourself.

An attacker can close the distance on you extremely fast. Studies have shown that a person can cover around twenty feet in 1.5 seconds. In that time, you can't even begin to unzip your purse to take out your weapon, even if you know you are being attacked. The same applies when going for a weapon in your car's glove compartment.

What happens when you are jumped, sucker punched or car jacked?

The odds of you using your concealed weapon in that situation are slim to none. Try getting to a weapon stored in your car when someone grabs you or sucker punches you through your window. Chances are slim that you'll be grabbing the weapon in the glove box.

Yes, anything is possible. But you shouldn't bet your life on any device except your own mind and body.

Unless you train with your weapon, safety device or cell phone in a high-stress environment, going over realistic scenarios on a weekly basis, it's unlikely you'll gain access to your device.

Even if you did get something out of your pocket or purse by luck, the chances of you being able to use the weapon or device effectively are slim to none without proper stress-inoculation training.

This also goes for dialing 911 on your phone. Do it in a high-stress situation when seconds matter or while you are being attacked. Try to dial, tell the operator your location, and describe the attacker and what's going on. It's extremely difficult, and while your focus is on the call, it is going to be difficult for you also to focus on what your attacker is doing.

Don't misunderstand what I am saying. Weapons, safety devices and cell phones can all help you survive, call for *help* or escape a situation. Just don't rely on them 100 per cent of the time. To be alert, your vision needs to be broad – your external focus extended and your critical focus not on one device.

Remember this important point: While you are focusing on your safety device, weapon or phone to help you escape harm, the attacker is focusing 110 per cent on attacking you and injuring you in the process.

Time and time again, it has been proven that your best weapon is your brain. Utilize your mind-to-body connection. In the heat of the moment, there is too much confusion, overwhelming stress, impact and pressure for you to be able to do much else.

Learn the proper tools and targets. Then rely on your mind to keep you safe.

Summary

This part of the book has completed your training with a look at the verbal and physical tools you can employ to escape a violent encounter. Where appropriate, you've learnt the strategies to defuse and de-escalate a situation. If you revisit Lily's story, you can see how she weighed up her options, and on the basis of how she felt about things and her reading of it all, chose to use tactics to defuse the situation. She chose to calm her employer down rather than escalate events, and this allowed her to remove him as an obstacle to the exit, enabling her to escape.

It is not always possible to do this, especially in a situation where you may have been surprised by someone who has the sole intent of doing you harm. Where avoiding or de-escalating a situation is not possible, then physical attack is the best offense. Strike hard, strike fast and strike first where at all possible.

I'd like to add a final word here on the limiting belief that it is only appropriate or "fair" to strike if you have been struck. If someone is intent on doing you harm and you recognize the precursors to physical attack, sometimes your only way out will be to strike first. You have to make the first move if at all possible. If they're intent on hurting you, your attacker is not going to be playing by any rules – following social conventions yourself could get you killed. Understand this key point – if you are struck first and struck hard, then it is going to lower your own performance. If your attacker's strike injures you badly, then you are going to be in a worse position to counter-attack, lowering your probability of escape. That is a fact. So work on the important idea of switching up the prey/predator mentality. Tap into your reason to prevail and go on the offense. Do whatever you can to escape and get to safety. Your life depends on it.

In this part of the book, we've gone through:

- How to act passive.

- How to act submissive.

- Verbal and physical engagement strategies to defuse and de-escalate a situation.

- The precursors to physical attack, so that you can be alert to the signals your attacker will give.

- The protective positions to take with your body, from which to guard yourself from injury and also launch your own attack.

- The combative tools to use to effectively harm your attacker in the form of body strikes.

- The targets to aim for on your attacker, and the best way to injure these.

- The idea that, at the end of the day, you need to rely on your mind, and your mind-body connection. This is your primary weapon.

- The idea that you have to keep it straightforward and simple. Whatever the circumstances, don't freeze. Breathe, think and move.

It's a lot to take in, which is why repetition is useful here. It's also why I have created the Quantum Academy. This is a community specifically for women just like yourself who want to learn a functional approach to personal safety in the privacy of your own home. The academy will give you everything you need to succeed: personal safety instructional videos, online courses, interviews with top experts, motivational videos and audios, and a private Facebook community where you can connect with likeminded people.

If I had to leave you with one piece of advice, it would be to remember that you *always* have options. Don't give up. And you will prevail against violence.

CONCLUSION

'Adapt what is useful, reject what is useless,
and add what is specifically your own.'

BRUCE LEE

T his book has been influenced by my long career as a strength and conditioning coach and self-protection instructor. It is the result of years of research and getting in the trenches with a variety of practical training methods from around the globe.

However, though I've passed on my guidance to keep you safe, and spoken from my experience, you must remember that no one personal safety system, art form or fighting method is necessarily the best.

When it comes to succeeding in life and protecting yourself during that journey, everything is individual. What works for someone else might not work for you in your specific situation or in the specific conflict you're faced with at one moment in time.

So don't worry about selecting the best tool for the moment from all of the information in your head — trust your gut and do what it tells you, taking comfort from the fact that you've been through your options and your mind/body will do what's best to keep you safe. Whatever works to bring you back home safe is the best tool, regardless of what it looks like to others.

As long as you keep your personal safety plan simple and practical under stress, then you don't have to worry about anything else. Develop the tools that can be used in high-stress situations for yourself, not someone else.

Your Personal Safety Plan

In the course of this book, we've gone through three keys to successful self-protection and covered different tools and strategies to improve your personal safety. This is the simplest way I know to help you stack the deck in your favor and keep yourself safe. This is your personal safety plan:

Prepare

- Understand that ninety per cent of training yourself to handle violence is mental. Survival is about mindset.

- Put yourself first, even if the idea seems selfish. Put the mask on yourself before doing anything else. You are a VIP, and your family, friends and loved ones need you.

- You Are It. Take responsibility for keeping yourself safe and see yourself as the first responder in any situation.

- Reprogram your brain to defeat and replace limiting beliefs through visualization exercises and positive affirmations.

- Understand that fear is there to help you. Fear is an alarm and fear is fuel.

- Tap into your reason to prevail. This is your purpose, your "why," the spark that ignites the jet fuel and gets your butt into gear.

- Form positive habits by taking small steps every day.

Avoid

- The best way to prevail against an attacker is to avoid a violent encounter.

- Look out for strangeness, not necessarily strangers.

- If you get that feeling that something just isn't right, it probably isn't. Trust your intuition.

- Being aware of something is passive. Being alert means being active and prepared to respond to something.

- You have to be alert for the people, places and things that could cause you harm as well as the people, places and things that can help you if needed.

- Concentrate on having broad vision and extended external focus rather than narrow vision and critical focus trained on some distraction, such as a cell phone, iPod, book or similar.

- Remember, an attacker chooses you. Watch your body language, make yourself a hard target, and de-select yourself.

Escape

- Our primary aim in every situation is getting away and reaching safety.

- Be proactive and become the predator.

- Engage verbally to defuse and de-escalate a situation where this is possible.

- Use passive and submissive tactics where appropriate.

- If all else fails and you have to engage physically, let your instincts do their work. They will cause you to compress or extend parts of your body to protect your vital areas (brain, eyes, throat), so you can think, breathe and move.

■ In a physical encounter: use gross motor tools, not fine motor skills; use closest tool on closest target; use soft tools for hard targets and hard tools for soft targets; and go for primary targets.

■ Strike first and strike hard. Go full throttle.

These are all the elements of a successful personal safety plan. All the tools and strategies and exercises in this book come down to these key principles of self-protection.

At this point, you may be asking: What next?

The answer is practice. Practice makes permanence. Please keep this book as your personal protection bible and go back over the ideas and exercises to reinforce the beliefs and hone the practices that will keep you safe.

To connect with like-minded people, join our exclusive community of members over at QuantumPersonalSafety.com. Here, you can further enhance your learning through access to articles, training videos, online courses and interviews with top safety experts.

You are part of a new movement of people thinking about self-protection in a different way, committed to personal safety – heart, mind and soul. Now you've put your safety first, you're in the position to share what you've learned, and you can help others protect themselves too. Thank you for reading.

BIBLIOGRAPHY

de Becker, Gavin (2002) *Fear Less*, Little, Brown and Company

de Becker, Gavin (2010) *The Gift of Fear*, Dell

Dimitri, Richard (2011) *Senshido: In Total Defense Of The Self*, Lulu

Dreeke, Robin (2013) *It's Not All About "Me": The Top Ten Techniques for Building Quick Rapport with Anyone*, People Formula

Hadnagy, Christopher (2010) *Social Engineering: The Art of Human Hacking*, Wiley

Hadnagy, Christopher (2014) *Unmasking the Social Engineer: The Human Element of Security*, Wiley

Horn, Sam (1997) *Tongue Fu! How to Deflect, Disarm, and Defuse any Verbal Conflict*, St Martin's Griffin

Larkin, Tim (2013) *Survive the Unthinkable*, Rodale

Larkin, Tim (2015) 'The Paradox of Violence', TEDxGrandForks (http://www.tedxgrandforks.com/)

Mann, Scott (2016) 'Rooftop Leadership', TEDxSantaBarbara (https://tedxsantabarbara.com/2016/scott-mann/)

Martin, Neal (2013) *Self Defense Tips Everyone Should Know*, Combative Mind Publications

Martin, Neal (2014) *Self Defense Solutions*, Combative Mind Publications

Miller, Rory (2008) *Meditations on Violence: A Comparison of Martial Arts Training & Real World Violence*, YMAA

Miller, Rory (2011) *Facing Violence: Preparing for the Unexpected*, YMAA

Miller, Rory (2015) *Conflict Communication: A New Paradigm in Conscious Communication*, YMAA

Morrison, Lee (2006) *A Complete Guide to Close Quarter Confrontation*, Volumes 1 & 2, New Breed

O'Dea, Gerard (2014) *Lone Worker Personal Safety Lessons in Protecting Health, Social and Community Workers*, Dynamis Insight

Robbins, Apollo (2013) 'The Art of Misdirection', TEDGLobal (https://www.ted.com/talks/apollo_robbins_the_art_of_misdirection)

Roberts, Chris (2010) *Danger Detection Strategies*, SAFE International

Thompson, Athena & Phil (2010) *Every Woman's Guide to Being Safe … For Life*, BookPal

Thompson, George (2007) *Verbal Judo: The Gentle Art of Persuasion*, Avon

ACKNOWLEDGEMENTS

First and foremost I want to thank my wife and my children for their unconditional love and support as well as my friends and family who have supported me every step of the way no-matter how long it took to get here.

We are never done learning and when the student is ready for the teacher he or she may appear. When you truly discover who you are deep down in your core you will start living the way you were meant to live.

I have had the honor and privilege of working with, learning from and researching some of the top strength and conditioning coaches and personal safety instructors in the world, as well as the best personal development coaches.

There are too many to list on this page but this book is a result of everything I have learned from the people I have worked with and the people I have researched. I owe all the mentors, teachers and coaches who have ever helped me in any way a big thank you!

In addition I would like to thank my editors from Grammar Factory, Jacqui, Carolyn and especially Sara, without you, this doesn't happen! I also want to thank my team at Morgan James Publishing who gave me a chance to prove myself, thank you!

ABOUT THE AUTHOR & QUANTUM PERSONAL SAFETY

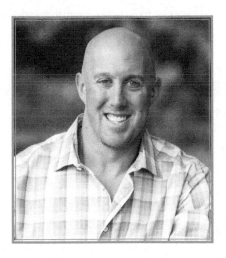

M Matt Tamas is a personal safety instructor and the founder of Quantum Personal Safety. He has spent the last eighteen years coaching people in personal safety, from lawyers, athletes and entrepreneurs to CEOs and moms.

Already a Certified Strength & Conditioning Specialist, Matt completed multiple personal safety certifications under coach Tony Torres, who developed the Functional Edge System of self-protection, while studying the best teaching techniques and training programs around the world with a multitude of instructors. Committed to personal development, Matt further undertook mentorships under executive coach Peter Sage and leadership expert Scott Mann. All his hard work has fed into his successful consulting business.

Bringing together everything he's learned throughout his personal safety career, Matt has designed QuantumPersonalSafety.com and the Quantum Academy for women to provide access to effective and practical personal safety instruction from your own home. Through joining the exclusive community of members, you can connect with like-minded people and further your learning through access to articles, training videos, online courses and interviews with top safety experts.

Matt's goal is to inspire women everywhere to take a proactive approach to prevailing against violence, and to engage in the simple steps to develop their own personal safety plan.

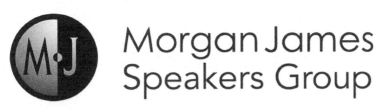

Morgan James
Speakers Group

We connect Morgan James published authors with live and online events and audiences whom will benefit from their expertise.

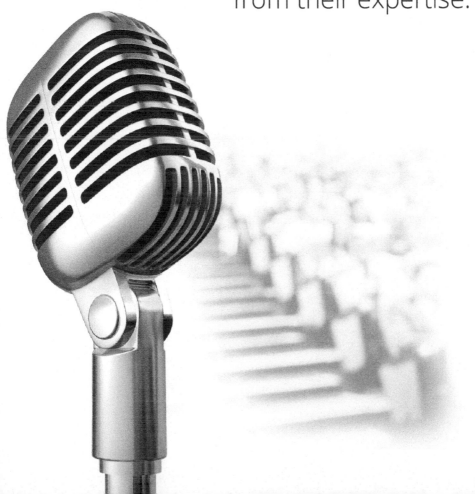

CPSIA information can be obtained
at www.ICGtesting.com
Printed in the USA
BVOW07s1215311017
499151BV00008B/99/P